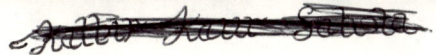

Contact lens optics

Contact lens optics

W. A. Douthwaite, MSc, PhD, FBCO, DCLP
Lecturer in Optometry, Bradford University

Butterworths
London Boston Durban Singapore Sydney Toronto Wellington

All rights reserved. No part of this publication may be reproduced
or transmitted in any form or by any means, including
photocopying and recording, without the written permission of
the copyright holder, applications for which should be addressed to
the Publishers. Such written permission must also be obtained
before any part of this publication is stored in a retrieval system of
any nature.

This book is sold subject to the Standard Conditions of Sale of
Net Books and may not be re-sold in the UK below the net price
given by the Publishers in their current price list.

First published 1987

© **Butterworth & Co. (Publishers) Ltd 1987**

British Library Cataloguing in Publication Data

Douthwaite, W. A.
  Contact lens optics.
  1. Contact lenses
  I. Title
  617.7'523   RE977.C6

ISBN 0-407-01330-X

Library of Congress Cataloging in Publication Data

Douthwaite, W. A. (William Arthur)
  Contact lens optics.
  Bibliography: p.
  Includes index.
  1. Contact lenses. 2. Optics, Physiological.
I. Title. [DNLM: 1. Contact Lenses. 2. Optics.
WW 355 D741c]
RE977.C6D68 1987   617.7'523   87-13783

ISBN 0-407-01330-X

Photoset by Latimer Trend & Company Ltd, Plymouth
Printed and bound in Great Britain by Anchor Brendon Ltd, Tiptree, Essex

Preface

This book could have been called *Notes on the Optics of Contact Lenses for Busy Contact Lens Practitioners* since an attempt has been made to cover the topic in the simplest possible way. The mathematics required for an understanding of the problems and their solutions is no more than very basic trigonometry and algebra. The author starts out by assuming that the reader may have forgotten everything ever learned in his or her optics and ophthalmic lenses lectures which may well have been attended decades ago. The first chapter deals with the fundamental principles and will hopefully revive fading memories. This then provides the foundation for solving the vast majority of contact lens optics problems that the practitioner may encounter in practice or the student may encounter during his or her undergraduate days.

The final chapter provides computer program listings that allow the contact lens practitioner to make use of information during the fitting procedure which would otherwise require resort to tables or tedious and often lengthy calculations. This being the case, many contact lens practitioners rely on their intuition when seeking a solution to, say, a fitting problem. The computer can be used to quantify the fitting relationship and to indicate, for example, the change in axial edge lift which occurs when a contact lens specification is altered. The results calculated by computer are sometimes surprising and this ensures that unnecessary or inappropriate changes to the lens specification are avoided.

I wish particularly to thank my colleague Jim Gilchrist for his help in organizing my computer programs into a more concise and efficient form; his contribution has been invaluable. I also wish to thank Michael Sheridan for reading the manuscript; his suggestions and encouragement have helped me, not only in writing this book but throughout my contact lens fitting career. I wish to thank Mrs J. Paley for typing the manuscript, and the staff of the Graphics Unit of the University of Bradford for their help with the diagrams.

Bradford   Bill Douthwaite

Contents

1 Basic visual optics   **1**

1.1 Lens power and vergence   1
1.2 Accommodation   3
1.3 Reduced thickness   10
1.4 Blur circles   11
1.5 Spectacle magnification   12
1.6 Relative spectacle magnification   19
1.7 Anisometropia   22
1.8 Convergence   23
1.9 Summary   26

2 The contact lens   **28**

2.1 The contact/fluid lens system   28
2.2 Calculation of surface radii   29
2.3 The relationship between front and back surfaces for a thick lens   31
2.4 Toric lens   34
2.5 Contact lens over-refraction using a lens with a BCOR different from that of the lens to be ordered   35
2.6 Contact lens over-refraction using a lens with an inappropriate BVP   37
2.7 Modifying anb existing lens   39
2.8 The BVP of scleral lenses produced by the impression techniques   46
2.9 Heine's scale   46

2.10　Edge and centre thickness　48
2.11　Edge lift　51
2.12　Aspheric contact lens surfaces　55
2.13　Offset or continuous bicurve lenses　58
2.14　Prismatic effects with contact lenses　61
2.15　Summary　64

3　Measurement of the cornea　66

3.1　The keratometer　66
3.2　The keratometer equation　66
3.3　Doubling　69
3.4　Mire image formation　71
3.5　The telecentric keratometer　72
3.6　One- and two-position instruments　75
3.7　Extending the range of measurement　76
3.8　The power scale　78
3.9　The keratometer used to check concave surfaces　80
3.10　Precautions　81
3.11　The topographic keratometer　81
3.12　The photokeratoscope　83
3.13　The pachometer　84

4　The cornea and contact lens combination　87

4.1　Corneal topography　87
4.2　Tear lens thickness and edge clearance　87
4.3　Calculation of TLT and edge clearance　88
4.4　Corneal astigmatism　89
4.5　Residual astigmatism　90
4.6　Back surface toric lenses　91
4.7　Front surface toric lenses　95
4.8　The fitting relationship on a toric cornea　99
4.9　Summary　105

5　Miscellaneous features　106

5.1　Bifocal contact lenses　106

5.2	The correction of the aphakic eye	114
5.3	The LVA telescope	120
5.4	Underwater lenses	125
5.5	Soft lenses	127
5.6	Radial thickness	136
5.7	Summary	139

6 Checking the lens specification — 140

6.1	The optical spherometer	140
6.2	The keratometer	145
6.3	The spherometer	149
6.4	The focimeter	151
6.5	The pachometer	159
6.6	The primary optic diameter of a scleral lens	160
6.7	Tolerances	162
6.8	Summary	174

7 Computer programs — 175

7.1	Effective power (lines 1000–1160)	176
7.2	Radius/power in air (lines 2000–2270)	177
7.3	Interface radius/power conversion (lines 3000–3240)	179
7.4	Front surface radius and FVP (lines 4000–4260)	180
7.5	Axial edge lift (lines 5000–5910)	182
7.6	Edge thickness and edge lift (lines 6000–6650)	186
7.7	BPOR for an offset lens (lines 7000–7300)	190
7.8	Aspheric surfaces (lines 8000–8230)	192
7.9	TLT and axial edge clearance (lines 8600–9990)	193
7.10	Lenticular edge thickness (lines 1500–1990)	200
7.11	The RC device (lines 2500–2660)	203
7.12	The menu (lines 10–390)	204
7.13	Lens thickness	205

References — 214

Index — 216

1 Basic visual optics

1.1 Lens power and vergence

In *Figure 1.1* the positive lens of power +1.00 D imparts convergence on the pencil of light rays from a point source at infinity. The vergence of light leaving the lens is +1.00 D. Since vergence is defined as the reciprocal of the distance (in metres) from a plane to the focal point, it follows that a point image is formed at a distance of 1 m from the lens. Also the vergence of light at plane A (50 cm from the focal point) will be +2.00 D, and the vergence of light at plane B will be +4.00 D. Thus it is obvious that any vergence relates to only one plane. In *Figure 1.1* the +1.00 D lens could be replaced by a +2.00 D lens at plane A or a +4.00 D lens at plane B. We can therefore state that the effective power of this lens at plane A is +2.00 D and the effective power of the lens at plane B is +4.00 D.

The distances measured in *Figure 1.1* are *from* the lens or the planes *to* the focussing point. In all three cases these distances are measured in the same direction as the direction of movement of the incident light and are in consequence considered as positive distances. They inevitably ensure that the pencil of light rays converge on one another. Convergence thus adopts the positive sign.

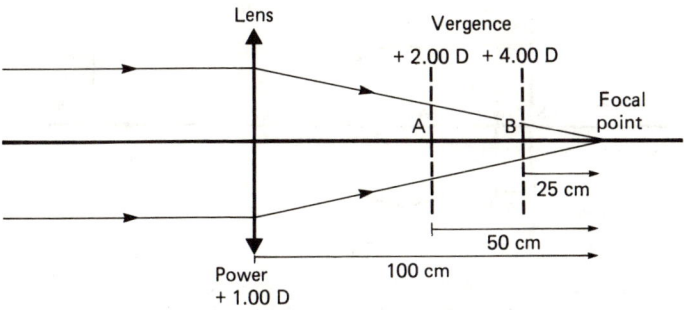

Figure 1.1. The relationship between distance and vergence.

2 Basic visual optics

In *Figure 1.2* an eye is corrected by a +10.00 D spectacle lens placed 15 mm in front of the cornea. Light rays leave this lens with a convergence of +10.00 D. If this lens corrects the eye for distance, the light rays must be converging on the far point of the eye since the far point can be defined as the point conjugate with the retina. Thus the principal focus of the lens F' must coincide with the far point of the eye M_R and the distance SM_R is 0.1 m. The effective power of the lens at C can be deduced as the reciprocal of the distance CM_R:

$$CM_R = 100 - 15$$
$$= 85 \text{ mm}$$

Thus the effective power of the spectacle lens at C is given by:

$$\frac{1}{0.085} = \frac{1000}{85}$$

$$= +11.76 \text{ D}$$

Thus a hyperope will need a contact lens which is more powerful than his or her spectacle lenses.

You will note in *Figure 1.2* that the measurement direction of the vertex distance is not indicated. This is intentional since it measures the distance between two optical components. In this particular problem we wished to determine the vergence required at C. The vertex distance measured from C is negative and consequently subtracted from SM_R. Readers who are confused by the sign convention need only look at the diagram to see that CM_R is less than SM_R and can therefore deduce that the vertex distance must be subtracted.

In *Figure 1.3* an eye is corrected by a −10.00 D spectacle lens at S:

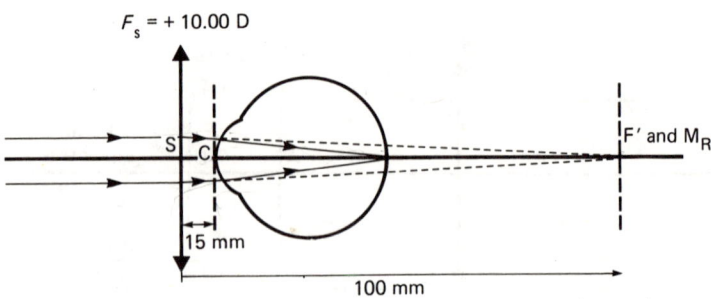

Figure 1.2. Spectacle correction of a 10.00 D hyperope. F_s is the power of the lens in the spectacle plane S. C represents the apex of the anterior cornea. M_R is the far point.

measurements made from CS

SMP + 65
     ___
      85

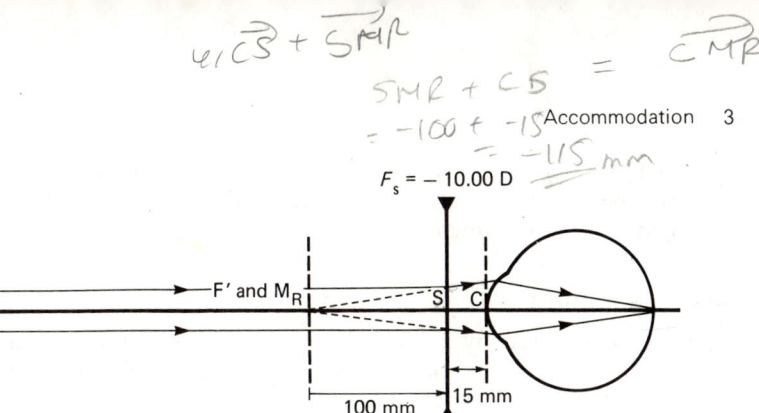

Figure 1.3. Spectacle correction of a 10.00 D myope. F_s is the power of the lens in the spectacle plane S. C represents the apex of the anterior cornea. M_R is the far point.

Far point distance $SM_R = \dfrac{1}{-10} \text{ m} = -100 \text{ mm}$

Here the distance from the lens to the focal point is measured *against the direction of incident light* and results in a divergent pencil of light rays.

The vertex distance measured from C is also a negative distance. The algebraic addition of these distances results in

$CM_R = -115 \text{ mm}$

Again the reader need only look at the diagram to deduce that CM_R is negative with a value of 115 mm.

Thus the effective power of the spectacle lens at C is

$\dfrac{1}{-0.115} = \dfrac{1000}{-115} = -8.70 \text{ D}$

A myope therefore will need a contact lens power which is less than his or her spectacle lenses.

From a clinical point of view this effect can be disregarded for spectacle lenses of power below ±4.00 D, since a 4.00 D spectacle lens at a typical vertex distance has an effective power at the cornea of around −3.75 D (myope) or +4.25 D (hyperope).

Chapter 7 includes a computer program which calculates the effective power at the eye of any spectacle lens at any vertex distance.

1.2 Accommodation

Clinically, accommodation is measured with a near-point rule and this is, strictly speaking, the spectacle accommodation. When deal-

4   Basic visual optics

ing with higher degrees of refractive error the spectacle accommodation may be an inadequate measurement. The problem is best illustrated by the following examples.

1.2.1 Example 1

A myope is corrected by a -6.00 D spectacle lens placed 14 mm from the cornea. What accommodation is exerted by the eye when looking at an object 40 cm from the spectacle plane:
  when using the spectacle correction?
  when corrected by a lens placed in the plane of the cornea?
This example asks for the accommodation exerted by the eye. Strictly speaking, therefore, we must deduce the ocular accommodation and this is referred to the principal refracting surface of the reduced eye. The cornea is only 1.67 mm in front of this plane. In order to simplify the treatment of the problem we will assume that the reduced surface and the cornea coincide. Strictly speaking we will be comparing spectacle accommodation with corneal accommodation. One other assumption that is made in this treatment is that the lenses involved are thin lenses. In order to clarify the difference between spectacle and ocular accommodation, a single diagram is drawn below with a light ray tracking through the distance path (accommodation relaxed) above the optical axis, and a light ray following the near path (accommodation active) below the optical axis.

1.2.1.1 The spectacle lens

As already mentioned we measure spectacle accommodation, i.e. we note (in dioptres) the reciprocal of the shortest distance at which a target can be clearly seen.
In *Figure 1.4*,

spectacle accommodation = vergence ① − vergence ③
vergence ① = 0.00 D   — since // light.
Since the distance OS is -40 cm
vergence ③ $= \dfrac{100}{-40} = -2.50$ D

∴ Spectacle accommodation = 2.50 D

What we are really saying here is that, at near, the incident vergence on the spectacle lens has become more negative than the distance vergence by 2.50 D. If the light rays are still focussed on the retina then the system must have become more positive (more converging)

Accommodation 5

thin lenses cornea coincides (handwritten)

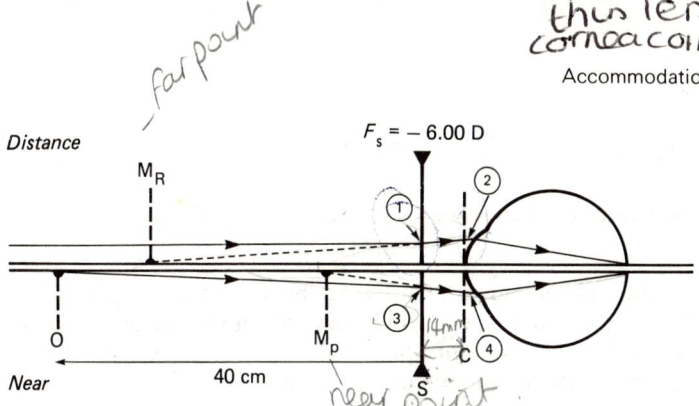

far point (handwritten, pointing to M_R)
near point (handwritten, pointing to S)

Figure 1.4. The spectacle correction in distance and near vision for a myope. O is the point object of interest in near vision. The numbers enclosed in circles represent vergences.

by this amount in the spectacle plane. This digression has nothing to do with the question but is included here for completeness.

The example asks for the accommodation exerted at the eye, and it does not take great powers of deduction to conclude that we need to concern ourselves with the incident vergences for distance and near, but at the eye and not the spectacle lens.

Thus

accommodation at the eye = vergence ② − vergence ④

Vergence ②

Distance $SM_R = \dfrac{100}{-6} = -16.67$ cm

Distance $CM_R = -16.67 - 1.4 = -18.07$ cm

∴ Vergence ② $= \dfrac{100}{-18.07} = -5.53$ D

(handwritten right side:)
$CMR = CS + SMR$
$= -1.4 + -\cancel{150}\ 166.7$
$= -5$
$= -180.7\quad \dfrac{100}{-18.07}$
$= -18.07$

Vergence ④

Incident light on the spectacle lens from the near object
$\qquad\qquad\qquad\qquad\qquad\qquad = -2.50$ D
$\qquad\qquad\qquad\qquad\qquad\qquad =$ vergence ③
Lens power $\qquad\qquad\qquad\qquad = -6.00$ D
∴ Emergent vergence from the spectacle lens $= -8.50$ D

∴ Distance $SM_p = \dfrac{100}{-8.5} = -11.76$ cm

Distance $CM_p = -11.76 - 1.4 = -13.16$ cm

$$\therefore \text{Vergence } ④ = \frac{100}{-13.16} = -7.60 \text{ D}$$

Accommodation at the eye = vergence ② − vergence ④
= 2.07 D

i.e. since the incident vergence at the eye becomes more negative by 2.07 D when changing from distance to near, the converging power of the eye must become more positive by the same amount if the light rays are to maintain a focus on the retina.

1.2.1.2 The contact lens

Figure 1.5 illustrates the arrangement for a correcting lens in the plane of the cornea. Once again,
  accommodation at the eye = vergence ② − vergence ④

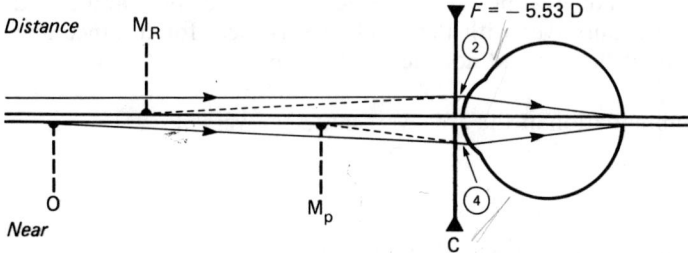

Figure 1.5. The contact lens correction in distance and near vision for a myope. The gap between the contact lens and the cornea is assumed to be thin and the contact lens is assumed to be a thin lens.

Vergence ②
  Contact lens refraction = vergence ② = −5.53 D

This was deduced in the previous section of this example and must be the back vertex power (BVP) of the correcting lens at C.

Vergence ④
  Distance OS = −40 cm

  Distance OC = −41.4 cm

$$\therefore \text{Incident vergence on the correcting lens} = \frac{100}{-41.4} = -2.42 \text{ D}$$

  Correcting lens BVP $\qquad\qquad\qquad\qquad = -5.53 \text{ D}$

∴ Emergent vergence = −7.95 D

This is vergence ④.

∴ Accommodation at the eye = 2.42 D

It is apparent from this example that myopes <u>must accommodate more with contact lenses</u> than when wearing spectacle corrections. It will be useful to repeat this exercise for the hyperope.

1.2.2 Example 2

A hyperope is corrected by a +6.00 D spectacle lens at a vertex distance of 14 mm. What accommodation is exerted by the eye when looking at an object 40 cm from the spectacle plane:
  when using the spectacle correction?
  when corrected by a lens in the plane of the cornea?

1.2.2.1 The spectacle lens

Figure 1.6 illustrates that once again the spectacle accommodation is 2.50 D, i.e. the same as the value for the myopic eye:
  Accommodation at the eye = vergence ② − vergence ④

Vergence ②
Since the lens power is +6.00 D, this must also be the emergent vergence from the lens at S.

∴ Distance $SM_R = \dfrac{100}{6} = 16.67$ cm

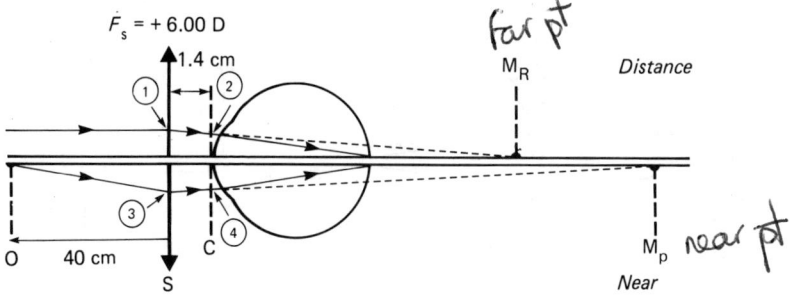

Figure 1.6. The spectacle correction in distance and near vision for a hyperope. O is the point object of interest in near vision. The numbers enclosed in circles represent vergences.

8   Basic visual optics

Distance $CM_R = 16.67 - 1.4 = 15.27$ cm

$\therefore$ Vergence ② $= \dfrac{100}{15.27} \quad = +6.55$ D

Vergence ④

Vergence ③ $= \dfrac{100}{-40} \quad = -2.50$ D

Lens power $\quad = +6.00$ D

$\therefore$ Emergent vergence from the lens at $S = +3.50$ D

$\therefore$ Distance $SM_p = \dfrac{100}{3.5} \quad = 28.57$ cm

Distance $CM_p = 28.57 - 1.4 \quad = 27.17$ cm

$\therefore$ Vergence ④ $= \dfrac{100}{27.17} \quad = 3.68$ D

Accommodation at the eye $= 6.55 - 3.68 = 2.87$ D

1.2.2.2 The contact lens

Vergence ②
Vergence ② $= +6.55$ D

This was deduced in the previous section of this example and it gives the BVP of the correcting lens at C.

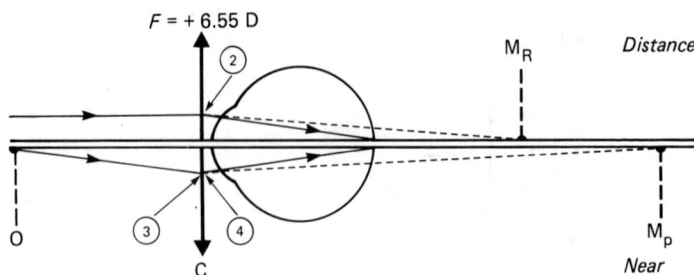

Figure 1.7. The contact lens correction in distance and near vision for a hyperope. The gap between the contact lens and the cornea is assumed to be thin and the contact lens is assumed to be a thin lens.

Vergence ④

Vergence ③ $= \dfrac{100}{-41.4} = -2.42$ D

Correcting lens BVP $= +6.55$ D

Vergence ④ $= +4.13$ D

Accommodation at the eye $= 6.55 - 4.13$

$\phantom{\text{Accommodation at the eye}}= 2.42$ D

N.B. This is the same value as that in the myopic eye when corrected by a contact lens.

1.2.3 Summary

A summary of the results is given in *Table 1.1*, which may help to clarify the picture.

The summary illustrates that, with contact lenses, both the myope and hyperope require the same accommodative effort at the eye. However, when wearing spectacles the effort is reduced for the myope but increased for the hyperope. Thus myopes need more accommodation for contact lens wear than for spectacle wear, hyperopes need less.

Table 1.1 Summary of results

Correction	Accommodation at the cornea
Myope—spectacle correction	2.07 D
Hyperope—spectacle correction	2.87 D
Myope—contact lens correction	2.42 D
Hyperope—contact lens correction	2.42 D

If the form and thickness of the lenses is taken into account by precise calculation, the results are found to be very similar for negative powers, with the discrepancy between ocular and spectacle accommodation increasing in the case of positive powers. However, the results produced on the basis of the presence of thin lenses may be taken as a close approximation.

1.3 Reduced thickness

In *Figure 1.8* an object O is emitting light rays which track towards the eye of an observer. Refraction occurs at the upper surface of the block so the light appears to be coming from O'. Thus the real thickness t of the block appears to have a value a as far as the observer is concerned.

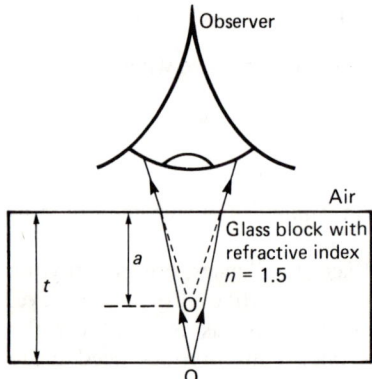

Figure 1.8. Refraction at a plane surface producing the apparent-depth effect.

The refractive index n of the glass can be deduced from the equation

$$n = \frac{\text{real depth}}{\text{apparent depth}} = \frac{t}{a}$$

$$\therefore a = \frac{t}{n}$$

Thus the apparent thickness is the actual thickness divided by the refractive index of the block. The value t/n is called the reduced thickness.

If we considered the vergences in *Figure 1.8* then the vergence of light from O at the upper surface of the block is $1/t$. The surface has no power. Therefore the emergent vergence is $1/t$. This is obviously incorrect.

The correct approach in these circumstances is to assume that the block has a reduced thickness t/n. We can then say that the vergence of light from O is n/t. The surface power is zero. Therefore the emergent vergence is n/t. This is obviously correct since we have just deduced that the apparent thickness is

$$a = \frac{t}{n}$$

Alternatively we could state that the light within the glass block has a reduced vergence of n/t. This once again results in an emergent vergence of n/t. Therefore either we consider a reduced thickness—this is the most useful approach when dealing with contact lenses—or we use the concept of reduced vergences—this is convenient for light rays travelling within the eye.

1.4 Blur circles

Figure 1.9 can be used to illustrate how to calculate blur circle diameters. The reduced vergence of the light rays emerging from **P** is n/f', i.e.

$$F = \frac{n}{f'}$$

$$\therefore f' = \frac{n}{F} = \frac{1}{60} \frac{4}{3} = 22.22 \text{ mm}$$

By similar triangles

$$\frac{\text{pupil diameter}}{f'} = \frac{\text{blur circle diameter}}{r'}$$

$$\therefore \text{Blur circle diameter} = \frac{\text{pupil diameter}}{f'} \times r'$$

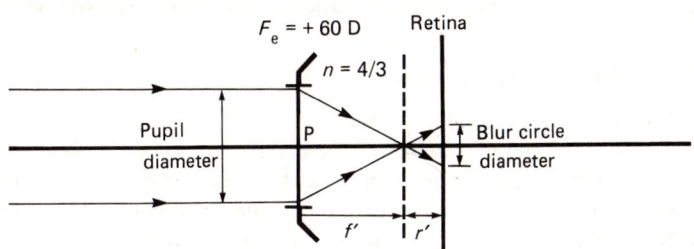

Figure 1.9. Blur circle formation on the retina of an axially myopic reduced eye of refractive power F_e and refractive index n.

1.5 Spectacle magnification

Using the reduced eye an object subtends a visual angle ω at P. The light ray in *Figure 1.10* is the principal light ray which, after refraction at P, can be used to determine the basic retinal image size. The assumption is made that the entrance and exit pupils coincide with the reduced surface P. The diagram illustrates that, for axial defects, the uncorrected basic retinal image size is largest for the myope and smallest for the hyperope. Since the image size variation is due to changes in axial length, it follows that in refractive defects the basic retinal image size does not alter with refractive error variations.

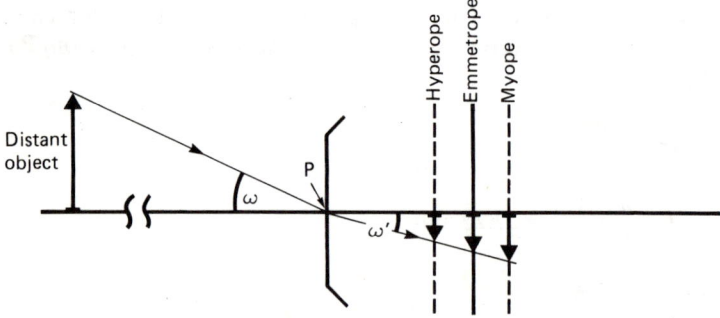

Figure 1.10. The basic retinal image size in uncorrected reduced eyes with axial ametropia. The light ray illustrated is the principal ray. The effect of the blur circles is not taken into account.

In order to calculate the actual retinal image size it is necessary to add one-half of a blur circle diameter to each end of the basic image, i.e. take the basic retinal image size and add one blur circle diameter.

1.5.1 The corrected eye

As shown in *Figure 1.11*, the spectacle lens which corrects the eye will produce an image (size h_1) of the distant object at the far point plane M_R. This image becomes the object for the corrected eye which will focus an image of height h_2 on the retina. In *Figure 1.11(a)* the correcting lens increases the visual angle $ω_0$ to $ω$ and this results in an increase in image size with correction. In *Figure 1.11(b)* the correcting lens decreases the retinal image size.

These diagrams illustrate that positive spectacle lenses make

look at visual optics.

13

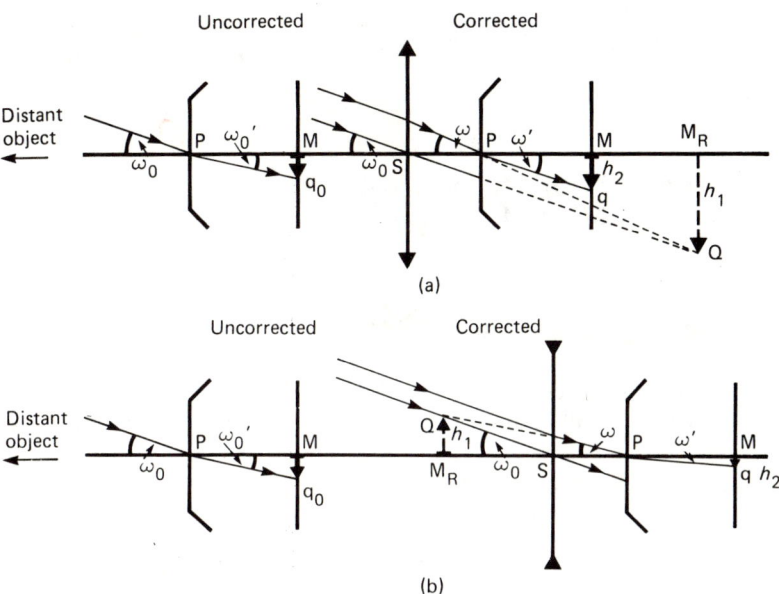

Figure 1.11. Change of retinal image size with the spectacle correction for (a) a hyperope and (b) a myope. The distant object subtends a visual angle ω_0 which is changed to ω by the spectacle lens. The spectacle lens produces an image (size h_1) of the distant object in the far-point plane of the eye (M_R). This image becomes the object for the eye.

things appear larger, and negative lenses have the opposite effect. Also the effect is increased by increasing the vertex distance.

Spectacle magnification is defined as retinal image size corrected divided by retinal image size uncorrected.

From *Figure 1.11(a)* and *(b)*

$$\text{Spectacle magnification} = \frac{Mq}{Mq_0}$$

but

$$\tan \omega' = \frac{Mq}{PM} \text{ and } \tan \omega'_0 = \frac{Mq_0}{PM}$$

14   Basic visual optics

$$\therefore \text{Spectacle magnification} = \frac{PM \tan \omega'}{PM \tan \omega'_0} = \frac{\tan \omega'}{\tan \omega'_0} = \frac{\tan \omega/n}{\tan \omega_0/n}$$

$$= \frac{\tan \omega}{\tan \omega_0}$$

$$\frac{\tan \omega}{\tan \omega_0} = \frac{M_R Q/PM_R}{M_R Q/SM_R} = \frac{M_R Q}{PM_R} \frac{SM_R}{M_R Q} = \frac{SM_R}{PM_R}$$

Thus

$$\text{spectacle magnification} = \frac{SM_R}{PM_R}$$

If the distances SM_R and PM_R are measured in metres their reciprocals will be the ocular and spectacle refraction respectively.

$$\therefore \text{Spectacle magnification} = \frac{1/PM_R}{1/SM_R}$$

$$= \frac{\text{ocular refraction}}{\text{spectacle refraction}}$$

This equation applies to hyperopia and myopia, both axial and refractive. A *contact lens* correction results in the equation

$$\text{contact lens magnification} = \frac{\text{ocular refraction}}{\text{contact lens refraction}}$$

With the positions of S and P almost coinciding, we can state that the spectacle magnification approximates to unity. Thus contact lenses do not alter the retinal image size significantly from that of the uncorrected eye. The foregoing is an approximation which arises from the use of the reduced eye. Strictly speaking, unity is achieved when the correcting lens is in the plane of the entrance pupil of the eye. The contact lens is likely to be 3 mm in front of the entrance pupil and it must be considered as a thick lens which is most certainly not flat. The fact that the lens is curved leads to displacement of the lens principal planes. Let us consider the influence of these factors.

1.5.2   The entrance pupil

In *Figure 1.12* the distant object which is situated on the axis of the system subtends an angle ω at the contact lens at C. If the eye were removed from the diagram this lens would form an image *h'* in the focal plane of the lens. The light ray in *Figure 1.12* passes through

Spectacle magnification 15

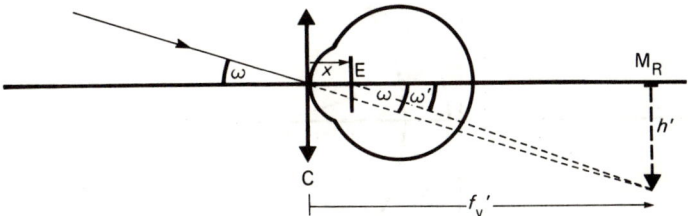

Figure 1.12. Spectacle magnification of a contact lens. The distant object subtends a visual angle ω. The correcting lens is placed at C which is *x*mm from E, the entrance pupil of the eye. The correcting lens produces an image (size *h'*) of the distant object in the far-point plane of the eye (M_R). This image becomes the object for the eye.

the optical centre of the lens; it therefore continues undeviated to emerge at an angle ω to the optical axis. However, when the eye is as shown in the diagram, *h'* becomes the object for the eye since it is in the far point plane M_R. Thus the corrected visual angle is ω' and

$$\text{spectacle magnification} = \frac{\omega'}{\omega}$$

$\tan \omega = \dfrac{-h'}{f_v'}$ (image is inverted) and $\tan \omega' = \dfrac{-h'}{f_v' - x}$

$$\therefore \text{Spectacle magnification} = \frac{-h'}{f_v' - x} \bigg/ \frac{-h'}{f_v'}$$

$$= \frac{f_v'}{f_v' - x}$$

$$\therefore \text{Spectacle magnification} = \frac{1}{1 - xF_v'}$$

where F_v' is the back vertex power (BVP) of the contact lens and *x* is the distance from the lens back vertex to the entrance pupil of the eye (in metres). The value $1/(1 - xF_v')$ is called the power factor of the lens.

1.5.3 The principal planes

In a thick lens the planes P and P' can be located by ray tracing as in *Figure 1.13*. The plane P' is of interest to the lens wearer since, for a parallel pencil of light coming from a distant object, the emergent light from the back surface of the lens follows the same track as that

16   Basic visual optics

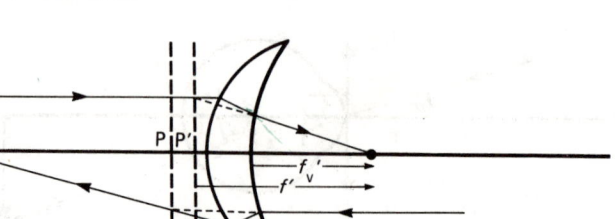

Figure 1.13. The principal planes (P and P') of a thick curved lens. f_v' is the back vertex focal length. f' is the equivalent focal length.

which emerges from a thin lens of focal length f' (equivalent focal length) placed in the plane P'. Thus the contact lens could be replaced by a thin lens at P'. The fact that the thick positive lens is curved results in P' being further from the eye and therefore increasing the spectacle magnification and hence the retinal image size.

1.5.3.1 The shape factor

If we assume in *Figure 1.14* that the contact lens is thin and of focal length f_v' then we can see that the image size at the far point of the eye is h_1. However, the thick curved contact lens will behave like an equivalent thin lens placed at P' of focal length f' (the equivalent focal length). Thus the contact lens actually produces an image size h_2. The ratio of these two image sizes is called the shape factor:

$$\text{Shape factor} = \frac{h_2}{h_1}$$

$$\tan \omega = \frac{-h_1}{f_v'} \text{ and } \tan \omega = \frac{-h_2}{f'}$$

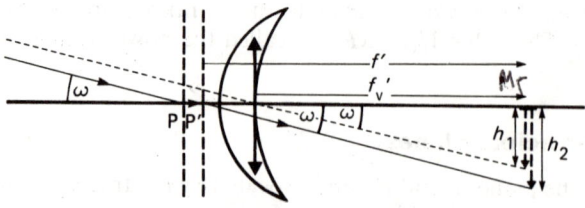

Figure 1.14. The shape factor. This diagram compares the image sizes produced by a thin flat lens and a thick curved lens with the same back vertex focal length from a distant object which subtends an angle ω at the lenses.

Spectacle magnification

$$\therefore \text{Shape factor} = \frac{-f' \tan \omega}{-f_v' \tan \omega} = \frac{f'}{f_v'}$$

If these distances are expressed in metres, then their reciprocals give the lens power in dioptres. Thus

$$\text{shape factor} = \frac{F_v'}{F'}$$

where F_v' is the back vertex power and F' is the power of the equivalent thin lens at P'.

For a single thick lens we can use the standard expressions

$$F_v' = \frac{F_1 + F_2 - (t/n)F_1 F_2}{1 - (t/n)F_1}$$

and

$$F = F_1 + F_2 - (t/n)F_1 F_2$$

where F_1 is the front surface power, F_2 is the back surface power and t/n is the reduced central thickness of the lens.

$$\therefore \text{Shape factor} = \frac{1}{1 - (t/n)F_1}$$

1.5.4 The fluid lens

We must now add to this the influence of the fluid lens. This can be

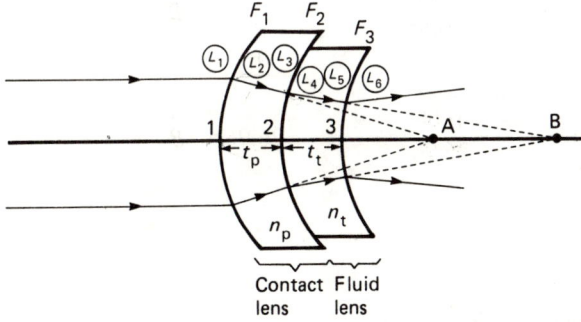

Figure 1.15. The shape factor for the contact lens and fluid lens in combination. The encircled letters represent vergences. F_1, F_2 and F_3 represent the powers of the front surface of the contact lens, the interface surface, and the posterior surface of the fluid lens respectively. t_p and t_t are the central thicknesses. n_p and n_t are the refractive indices of the contact lens and fluid lens respectively.

18 Basic visual optics

done by calculating the equivalent power of the contact lens and fluid lens in combination. Suppose in *Figure 1.15*

$F_1 = +54.69$ D, $F_2 = -19.25$ D, $F_3 = -43.08$ D

$t_p = 0.6$ mm, $t_t = 0.4$ mm, $n_p = 1.490$, $n_t = 1.336$

Using the 'step along' method which converts vergences to distances, alters the distances and converts them back to vergences we have:

Vergence (D)		Distance (mm)
$L_1 = 0.00$		
$F_1 = +54.69$		
$L_2 = +54.69 \longrightarrow$	$\dfrac{1000}{54.69}$	$\longrightarrow 18.28 = 1A$
		$-0.4 = t_p/n_p$
$L_3 = +55.93 \longleftarrow$	$\dfrac{1000}{17.88}$	$\longleftarrow 17.88 = 2A$
$F_2 = -19.25$		
$L_4 = +36.68 \longrightarrow$	$\dfrac{1000}{36.68}$	$\longrightarrow 27.26 = 2B$
		$-0.3 = t_t/n_t$
$L_5 = +37.09 \longleftarrow$	$\dfrac{1000}{26.96}$	$\longleftarrow 26.96 = 3B$
$F_3 = -43.08$		
$L_6 = -5.99$		

Again the shape factor is $\dfrac{F'_v}{F'}$ and

$L_6 = F'_v$

F' can be deduced from the thick lens equation

Relative spectacle magnification 19

$$F = \frac{L_2 L_4 L_6}{L_3 L_5} = \frac{(+54.69)(+36.68)(-5.99)}{(+55.93)(+37.09)}$$
$$= -5.79 \text{ D}$$

$$\therefore \text{Shape factor} = \frac{-5.99}{-5.79} = 1.035$$

1.5.5 Total spectacle magnification

The total spectacle magnification must be the product of spectacle magnification (assuming thin lenses) and the shape factor of the system.

Total spectacle magnification = power factor × shape factor

$$= \frac{1}{1 - xF_v'} \times \text{shape factor}$$

where x is the distance from the contact lens back vertex to the entrance pupil of the eye (in metres) and F_v' is the contact lens BVP (in dioptres).

Calculations reveal that scleral contact lenses produce retinal images that are larger than those produced by corneal lenses, owing to the scleral lens possessing a larger shape factor; this arises in the main from the greater central thickness of the scleral lens.

1.6 Relative spectacle magnification

Relative spectacle magnification is defined as

$$\frac{\text{size of retinal image in corrected ametropic eye}}{\text{size of retinal image in standard emmetropic eye}}$$

1.6.1 Size of image in corrected ametropic eye

In *Figure 1.16*, consider light incident on F_1 from a distant object; then

$$L_2 = L_1 + F_1$$
$$L_3 = \frac{L_1 + F_1}{1 - d(L_1 + F_1)}$$

and

$$L_4 = \frac{L_1 + F_1}{1 - d(L_1 + F_1)} + F_e$$

20 Basic visual optics

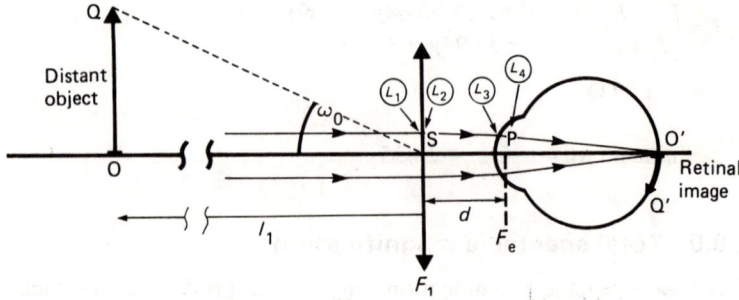

Figure 1.16. The retinal image size in the corrected eye. The encircled letters represent vergences. The distant object OQ subtends a visual angle ω_0 and produces a retinal image O'Q'. F_1 is the power of the spectacle lens. F_e is the power of the eye. d is the vertex distance.

If we take the general equation for magnification as

$$\text{magnification} = \frac{L_1}{L_2}\frac{L_3}{L_4}$$

and substitute the values above in this equation we conclude that

$$\text{magnification} = \frac{L_1}{L_1 + F_1 + F_e - dL_1F_e - dF_1F_e}$$

But

image size = object size × magnification

and

$$\text{object size} = \omega_0 l_1 = \frac{\omega_0}{L_1}$$

$$\therefore \text{Image size} = \frac{\omega_0}{L_1} \frac{L_1}{L_1 + F_1 + F_e - dL_1F_e - dF_1F_e}$$

$$= \frac{\omega_0}{L_1 + F_1 + F_e - dL_1F_e - dF_1F_e}$$

If the object is considered to be at infinity then $L_1 = 0$.

$$\therefore \text{Image size} = \frac{\omega_0}{F_1 + F_e - dF_1F_e}$$

1.6.2 Size of image in the standard emmetropic eye

In *Figure 1.17*

$$\omega_0' = \frac{h'}{f_0'} \quad \therefore h' = f_0'\omega_0'$$

Relative spectacle magnification 21

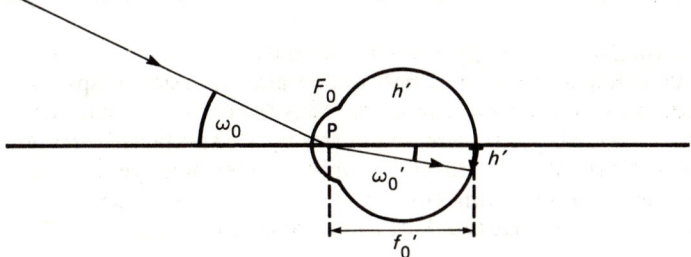

Figure 1.17. The retinal image in the standard emmetropic eye. The distant object subtends a visual angle ω_0 at the reduced surface P of power F_0. The refractive index of the eye is n' and the retinal image size is h'.

But
$$f'_0 = \frac{n'}{F_0} \quad \therefore h' = \frac{n'}{F_0}\omega'_0$$
But
$$\omega'_0 = \frac{\omega_0}{n'} \quad \therefore h' = \frac{\omega_0}{F_0}$$

1.6.3 Relative spectacle magnification

If we now substitute the expressions for the two retinal image sizes into the relative spectacle magnification definition we deduce that

$$\text{relative spectacle magnification} = \frac{\omega_0/(F_1 + F_e - dF_1F_e)}{\omega_0/F_0}$$

$$= \frac{F_0}{F_1 + F_e - dF_1F_e}$$

1.6.4 Axial ametropia

In axial ametropia
$$F_e = F_0$$

$$\therefore \text{Relative spectacle magnification} = \frac{F_0}{F_1 + F_0 - dF_1F_0}$$

$$= \frac{1}{1 + F_1(f_0 - d)}$$

If d equals f_0 then the relative spectacle magnification is unity, i.e. the corrected image size is the same as that of the standard emmetropic eye.

d is usually less than f_0. There $f_0 - d$ results in a positive value. If the eye is hyperopic F_1 will be positive and the relative spectacle magnification will be less than unity. Thus the corrected image in an axially hyperopic eye is increased in size by the spectacle correction but it is still smaller than the image in the emmetropic eye. In axially myopic eyes the minifying correction still leaves an image which is larger than that of the standard emmetropic eye.

1.6.5 Refractive ametropia

Since the image size in the corrected eye is equal to the image size in the standard emmetropic eye (both have the same axial lengths) then the spectacle magnification must be equal to the relative spectacle magnification. Therefore the relative spectacle magnification is greater than unity in hyperopia and less than unity in myopia.

1.7 Anisometropia

Correction of an anisometrope with contact lenses results in the obvious advantage of a correcting lens that moves with the eye. Thus the prismatic effects that result from looking through an area of a correcting lens eccentric to its optical centre are minimized. Prism induced by lens decentration produces relative vertical and horizontal prism in the eyes of anisometropes with the relative vertical prism being particularly troublesome. However, we must also consider the effects of changes in retinal image size and this will be influenced by the type of ametropia (axial or refractive).

1.7.1 Refractive anisometropia

In refractive anisometropia the uncorrected retinal image size will be the same in the two eyes. Positive correcting lenses will magnify, and negative correcting lenses will minify, the retinal image. Thus correcting lenses will induce an image size disparity which may result in binocular vision problems. A pair of contact lenses will induce a much smaller change than a pair of spectacle lenses. Therefore a contact lens correction appears to be the more satisfactory of the two alternatives.

1.7.2 Axial anisometropia

In axial anisometropia the uncorrected myopic eye will possess a larger than normal retinal image size which will be reduced by a correcting spectacle lens. However, the relative spectacle magnification will still be greater than unity, i.e. the correcting lens is only partially successful in returning the image to a normal size. A contact lens will alter the image size less than a spectacle lens and so we can see that the large uncorrected image will be returned to a more normal size by a spectacle lens, with the contact lens having a less pronounced influence. The axially hyperopic eye will also be better corrected by a spectacle lens since the small uncorrected retinal image will be magnified. It therefore appears on strictly optical grounds that the spectacle correction reduces the disparity between the image sizes in the two eyes more effectively than a contact lens correction.

However, suggestions have been made in the past that an axially myopic eye will have its retina stretched over a large area (owing to the larger than normal size of the eye) and this may increase the receptor spacing. If this notion is accepted then a particular object at a particular distance may, for example, produce an image on the uncorrected eye retina which subtends five receptors. In the axially hyperopic eye where the receptors are more densely packed, the same object will produce a smaller uncorrected image which could well still stimulate five receptors. The neural image size in these two eyes is thus identical and an ideal correction would be one that did not alter the uncorrected retinal image sizes. Thus a contact lens correction would be preferable to a spectacle lens correction.

Anisometropia is more likely to be axial than refractive and the foregoing indicates unfortunately that the fundamentals have not yet been unequivocally resolved. The only thing that can be stated with some certainty is that, if an anisometrope has comfortable binocular vision with a spectacle correction, he or she can expect to encounter adaptation problems when transferring to contact lenses.

A recent study by Winn *et al.* (1986) has concluded that all anisometropes are better corrected by contact lenses to minimize aniseikonic effects. They propose that in the case of the axial anisometrope the receptive field sizes compensate for the difference in retinal image size and this results in congruous cortical images.

1.8 Convergence

Let us take as an example an uncorrected myope observing a letter at a distance of 33.3 cm. The eyes are converging as shown in *Figure 1.18*. It can be seen that the convergence required is greater for larger pupillary distances (PDs). Let us assume that the PD is 60 mm. The convergence unit most commonly encountered is the prism dioptre (Δ) which is defined as a deviation of 1 cm in 1 m, i.e. the angle of deviation in prism dioptres is the tangent of the angle multiplied by 100. Therefore in *Figure 1.18* the convergence in prism dioptres is

$$\frac{30}{333} 100 = 9 \, \Delta$$

It can also be noted that the angle of covergence could be stated in metre angles. The metre angle is defined as the reciprocal of the distance in metres. In *Figure 1.18*

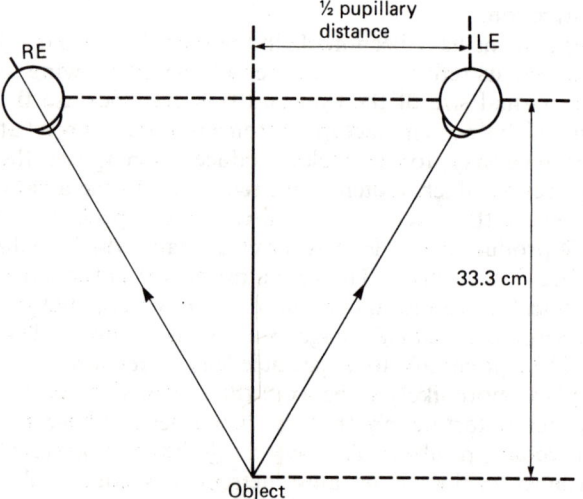

Figure 1.18. Convergence onto a point object 33.3 cm from a pair of uncorrected eyes.

$$\text{convergence in metre angles} = \frac{1}{1/3} = 3$$

∴ Convergence in prism dioptres = ½ PD (cm) × metre angle

If the myope is corrected by contact lenses and we assume that the lenses remain in a central position on convergence, then the myope will still require 9 Δ convergence in each eye in order to view the object of interest at 33.3 cm.

Convergence 25

In *Figure 1.19* the myope is corrected by −6.00 DS spectacle lenses 25 mm in front of the centres of rotation, with these lenses centred for the distance PD of 60 mm. When the eyes converge to look at the object 33.3 cm away the visual axes pass through a point on the nasal side of the optical centre of both lenses. This introduces a base in prism which reduces the convergence required.

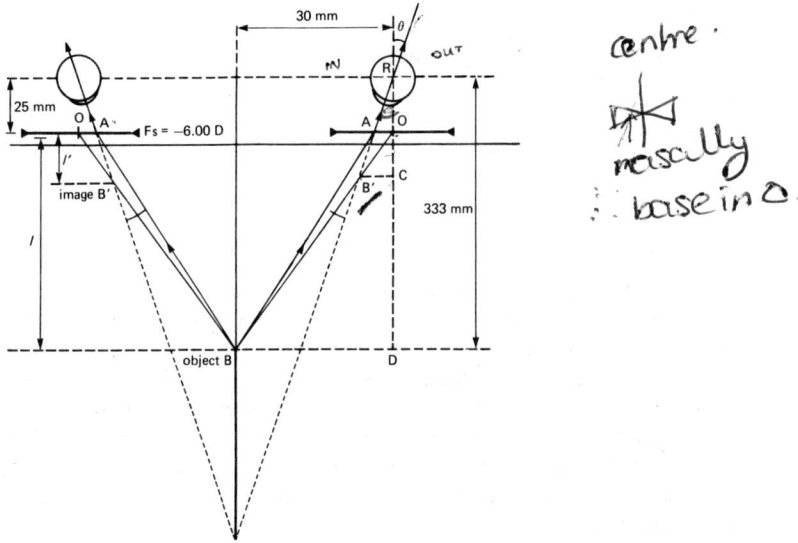

Figure 1.19. Convergence onto a point object 33.3 cm from a pair of corrected myopic eyes. The spectacle lens power is −6.00 D situated 25 mm in front of the centres of rotation of the eyes. The spectacle lenses have their optical centres (O) set at the distance PD of 60 mm.

The −6.00 DS lens will produce an image B′ of the object B and this image must lie on the line which joins the object to the optical centre of the lens O.

Object distance $l = -333 + 25 = -308$ mm

giving an object vergence of

$$\frac{1000}{-308} = -3.25 \text{ D}$$

Lens power = −6.00 D

∴ Image vergence = −9.25 D

giving an image distance

$$l' = \frac{1000}{-9.25} = -108.11 \text{ mm}$$

From *Figure 1.19*, in the triangle BOD

$$\frac{B'C}{BD} = \frac{l'}{l}$$

$$\therefore B'C = \frac{108.11}{308} 30 = 10.53 \text{ mm}$$

$$\tan \theta = \frac{B'C}{CR} = \frac{10.53}{133.11} = 0.0791$$

Convergence of each eye in prism dioptres = $\tan \theta \times 100$

$\therefore$ Each eye converges 7.91 Δ

Thus the 9 Δ of convergence required in each eye when uncorrected or corrected by a well centred contact lens is reduced by just over 1 Δ when the eye is corrected by the spectacle lens.

We can conclude that negative spectacle lenses reduce the convergence required. Positive spectacle lenses centred for distance vision will require an increase of convergence over that required when uncorrected. Therefore a myope wearing contact lenses requires more convergence than when wearing spectacles, and vice versa for the hyperope.

It will be recalled that myopes accommodate more, hyperopes accommodate less, when wearing contact lenses instead of a spectacle correction. This means that the accommodation/convergence relationship is only minimally disturbed.

1.9 Summary

- Vergence in dioptres is the reciprocal of distance in metres and vice versa.
- Convergence is positive, divergence is negative. A positive vergence will be accompanied by a positive distance.
- Hyperopes need more powerful contact lenses. Myopes need more powerful spectacle lenses.
- Clinically the effective power of a spectacle lens at the eye is of no consequence under ± 4.00 D.
- The uncorrected basic retinal image size is determined by the axial

length of the eye. The larger eye produces a larger retinal image.
- Positive spectacle lenses increase the retinal image size. Negative lenses decrease the retinal image size. The effect is more pronounced with large vertex distances.
- In axial ametropia the increase in retinal image size due to a positive spectacle lens produces an image which is still smaller than that of an emmetropic eye. Corrected axial myopes possess retinal image sizes which are larger than those of the emmetrope.
- Hyperopes require less accommodation and less convergence, having transferred to contact lenses from spectacle lenses. Myopes accommodate more and converge more with contact lenses.

2 The contact lens

OS = overall size

2.1 The contact/fluid lens system

When a contact lens is placed on the eye the tear fluid trapped between the contact lens and the cornea forms a fluid lens as shown in *Figure 2.1(a)*. However, it is often convenient to 'pretend' that the system is as shown in *Figure 2.1(b)* where the contact lens, fluid lens and cornea are separated by two infinitely thin air films. In these circumstances we can readily see that a contact lens with a back vertex power (BVP) of -2.00 D in air will correct a 2.00 D myope when placed in contact with the eye (this assumes that the fluid lens is afocal).

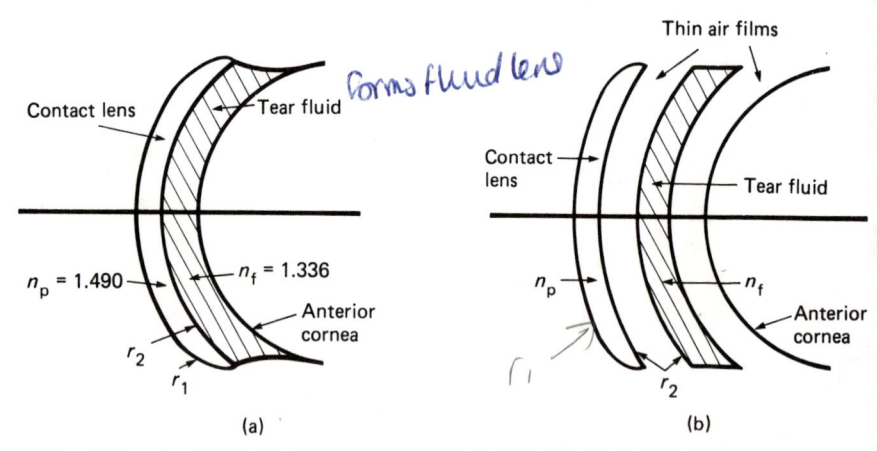

Figure 2.1. The contact lens on the eye. n_p is the refractive index of the plastic (1.490), n_f is the refractive index of the fluid (1.336) and r_2 is the radius of curvature of the interface.

Let us assume that the contact lens back central optic radius (BCOR) r_2 is 7.80 mm, with a refractive index n_p of 1.490. The tear fluid refractive index n_f is assumed to be 1.336.

In *Figure 2.1(a)* the power of the contact lens/fluid lens interface is

$$\frac{n_f - n_p}{r_2 \text{ (metres)}} = \frac{-154}{7.8}$$

$$= -19.74 \text{ D}$$

Thus light rays undergo a vergence change of -19.74 D as they cross the contact lens/fluid lens interface.

There is a computer program in Chapter 7 which performs this calculation for media of any refractive index.

In *Figure 2.1(b)* the power of the back surface of the contact lens in air is

$$\frac{1 - n_p}{r_2 \text{ (metres)}} = \frac{-490}{7.8}$$

$$= -62.82 \text{ D}$$

The power of the front surface of the fluid lens in air is

$$\frac{n_f - 1}{r_2 \text{ (metres)}} = \frac{336}{7.8}$$

$$= +43.08 \text{ D}$$

In *Figure 2.1(b)* the light rays undergo a total vergence change of $-62.82 + 43.08 = -19.74$ D as they leave the contact lens and enter the fluid lens.

Clearly the presence of an infinitely thin film of air has no effect on the path of the light rays through the system, and provided the fluid lens has no power (as is the case in an alignment fitting) then the power of the contact lens in air should equal the ocular refraction.

2.2 Calculation of surface radii

Contact lens surfaces are of very short radius and therefore very high power. We must always consider contact lenses as thick lenses. In practice an optometrist decides on a suitable back central optic radius (BCOR) in order to ensure an acceptable fit. The optometrist goes on to perform a contact lens over-refraction in order to deduce the contact lens BVP to be ordered. The contact lens laboratory must, in manufacturing the lens, provide it with the correct BCOR

30   The contact lens

[handwritten: this is L_6 since // light enters the eye.]

and deduce the front surface radius required to provide the BVP requested. The calculation of front surface radius in these circumstances may best be illustrated by the following example.

An optometrist decides that a fitting set lens with a BCOR of 8.00 mm provides a good fit. The trial set lens has a BVP of −1.00 D. The over-refraction results in a +2.00 DS in the refractor head. What front surface radius is required for this lens if the final centre thickness is 0.6 mm?

Since the lens in the refractor head is less than 4.00 D we can ignore the effect of vertex distance. Therefore the contact lens BVP to be ordered is −1.00 + 2.00 = +1.00 D.

If the central thickness t is 0.6 mm, and the refractive index n for the contact lens material is 1.490, then the reduced thickness t/n is 0.4 mm (to two significant figures). In *Figure 2.2* the vergence L_4 is the BVP of the contact lens (+1.00 D).

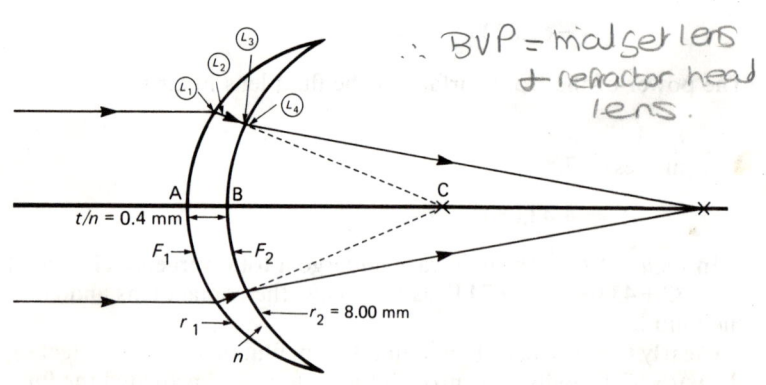

[handwritten: ∴ BVP = trial set lens + refractor head lens.]

Figure 2.2. Deduction of the front surface radius. The vergences are enclosed in circles.

It was decided to abandon the accepted sign convention using L_1, L_1', L_2, L_2', etc. since it is the author's experience that this leads to errors arising from neglecting to include the dash or mixing L_1 with L_1', for example, because of their similarity

We can use the step along method to work through the system to deduce the front surface radius as follows:

Contact lens back surface power

$$F_2 = \frac{1-n}{r_2 \text{ (metres)}} = \frac{-490}{8} = -61.25 \text{ D}$$

Vergence (D)			Distance (mm)	
$L_4 =$	$+1.00$	$L_2 = f_1 + \ell_1$	$L_a = f_2 + l_3$	
$F_2 =$	-61.25			
$L_3 =$	$+62.25$	$\dfrac{1000}{62.25}$	$\rightarrow 16.06 = BC$	
			$0.4 = t/n$	
$L_2 =$	$+60.75 \leftarrow$	$\dfrac{1000}{16.46}$	$16.46 = AC$	
$L_1 =$	00.00			

$\therefore F_1 = +60.75$

$$r_1 = \frac{n-1}{F_1} = \frac{490}{60.75} = 8.07 \text{ mm}$$ ✓

The deduction of L_3 may not be immediately obvious until we look at the lens. An incident vergence of $+62.25$ D on a surface of power -61.25 D will result in an emergent vergence of $+1.00$ D. Indeed it is good practice to cross check a result in this way before proceeding further. The point to remember is that the algebraic addition of the incident vergence and the surface power gives the emergent vergence. That is

$L_3 + F_2 = L_4$

$\therefore L_3 = L_4 - F_2$

2.3 The relationship between front and back surfaces for a thick lens

In the last example the step along method was used to determine the front surface radius of the contact lens which was assumed to be thick. An alternative approach to this problem is to assume initially that the lens is thin and proceed with calculating the front surface radius on that basis. The radius is then finally adjusted by adding a correction factor which takes the lens thickness into account. This approach is quicker than the step along method. The correction factor is most conveniently derived by considering an afocal lens as described below.

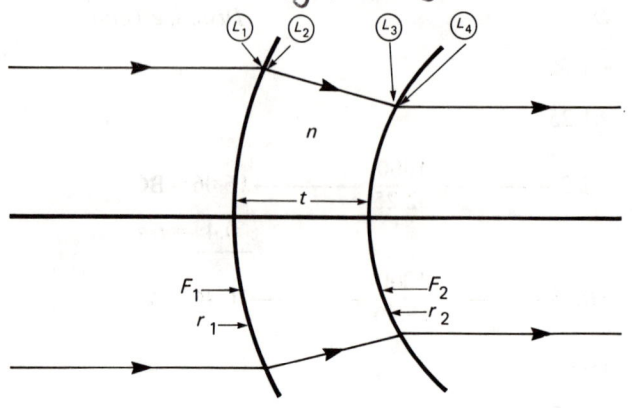

32 The contact lens ~light incident & light emergent = parallel. Afocal lens.~

Figure 2.3. An afocal thick lens. F_1 and F_2 are the surface powers arising from surface radii of r_1 and r_2 respectively, t is the central thickness, n is the refractive index.

In *Figure 2.3*

$$L_1 = 0.00, \quad L_2 = F_1, \quad L_3' = \frac{F_1}{1-(t/n)F_1}$$

and

$$L_4 = \frac{F_1}{1-(t/n)F_1} + F_2 = 0.00 \text{ for an afocal lens}$$

$$\therefore F_2 = -\left(\frac{F_1}{1-(t/n)F_1}\right) \text{ but } F_2 = \frac{1-n}{r_2}$$

$$\therefore \frac{1-n}{r_2} = -\left(\frac{F_1}{1-(t/n)F_1}\right)$$

$$-\left(\frac{n-1}{r_2}\right) = -\left(\frac{F_1}{1-(t/n)F_1}\right) \quad \text{~subst } F_1 = \frac{n-1}{r_1}.~$$

$$\therefore \frac{n-1}{r_2} = \frac{(n-1)/r_1}{1-(t/n)\{(n-1)/r_1\}}$$

Divide each side by $n-1$ to get

The relationship between front and back surfaces for a thick lens

$$\frac{1}{r_2} = \frac{1/r_1}{1-(t/n)\{(n-1)/r_1\}}$$

$$\therefore r_2 = \frac{1-(t/n)\{(n-1)/r_1\}}{1/r_1} = r_1\left\{1-\frac{t}{n}\left(\frac{n-1}{r_1}\right)\right\}$$

$$r_2 = r_1 - \frac{t}{n}(n-1) = r_1 - \frac{n-1}{n}t$$

and

$$r_1 = r_2 + \frac{n-1}{n}t$$

For a thin afocal lens

$$r_1 = r_2$$

For a thick afocal lens

$$r_1 = r_2 + \frac{n-1}{n}t$$

i.e. the front surface must be flatter than the back by an amount $\{(n-1)/n\}t$ which approximates to one-third of the lens centre thickness.

This relationship, derived by Bennett (1985), can be applied to thick powered lenses as shown by repeating the previous example which requested calculation of the front surface radius.

In *Figure 2.4* we commence the calculation with the assumption that the lens is thin:

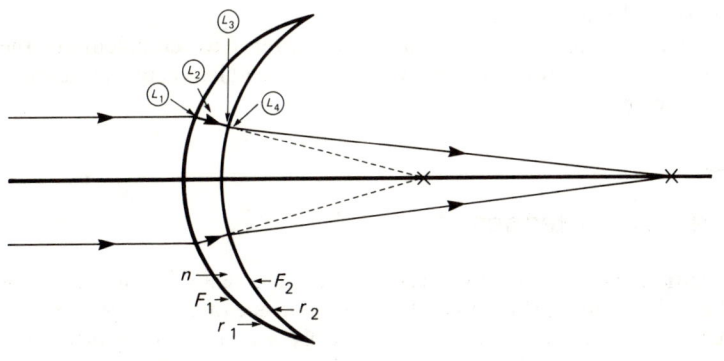

Figure 2.4. Deduction of front surface radius for a thin lens.

$$F_2 = \frac{1-n}{r_2} = \frac{-490}{8} = -61.25 \text{ D}$$

$L_4 = +1.00 \text{ D}$

$F_2 = -61.25 \text{ D}$

$L_3 = +62.25 \text{ D}$

Since the lens is thin this vergence is not only the incident vergence on the back surface but also the emergent vergence L_2 from the front surface of the lens, i.e.

$L_2 = +62.25 \text{ D}$

$L_1 = \underline{00.00 \text{ D}}$

$\therefore F_1 = +62.25 \text{ D}$

$$r_1 = \frac{n-1}{F_1} = \frac{490}{62.25} = 7.87 \text{ mm}$$

But the lens is thick so we must add a correction factor of $\{(n-1)/n\}t$ to this front surface radius:

$$\frac{n-1}{n}t = \frac{0.490}{1.490}\,0.6 = 0.2 \text{ mm}$$

Therefore, for a thick lens,

$r_1 = 7.87 + 0.2 = 8.07 \text{ mm}$

It will be noted that this is in agreement with the answer obtained by the step along method.

There is a computer program in Chapter 7 which calculates the front surface radius when the BVP, BCOR and lens central thickness are known.

2.4 Toric lenses

A toric contact lens introduces no extra problems for deduction of the radii of one surface when the other surface radii, lens power, and centre thickness are known. It is simply a matter of regarding the two principal meridians as separate lenses so that the calculation is performed as above for the first meridian and repeated for the second.

2.5 Contact lens over-refraction using a lens with a BCOR different from that of the lens to be ordered

Occasionally the contact lens practitioner will not have a contact lens of the desired BCOR for the purpose of over-refracting the patient. In these circumstances a contact lens with a BCOR as near as possible to that to be ordered can be used and the final BVP adjusted to compensate for the fact that the over-refraction was performed with a contact lens of BCOR different from that of the ordered lens.

This is best illustrated by the following example.

A trial lens with a BCOR of 8.00 mm and BVP of -2.00 D is worn by an eye and an over-refraction is performed. When the end point is reached the lens in the refractor head is $+0.50$ DS. We intend to order a lens with a BCOR of 8.25 mm. What BVP should be ordered for this lens?

In *Figure 2.5* we see the contact lens that would have been ordered if the BCOR was to remain unchanged at 8.00 mm. In this case the BVP requested would be $-2.00 + 0.50 = -1.50$ D. Thus $L_4 = -1.50$ D. This is the vergence of light in the thin air film which is equal to the lens BVP in air.

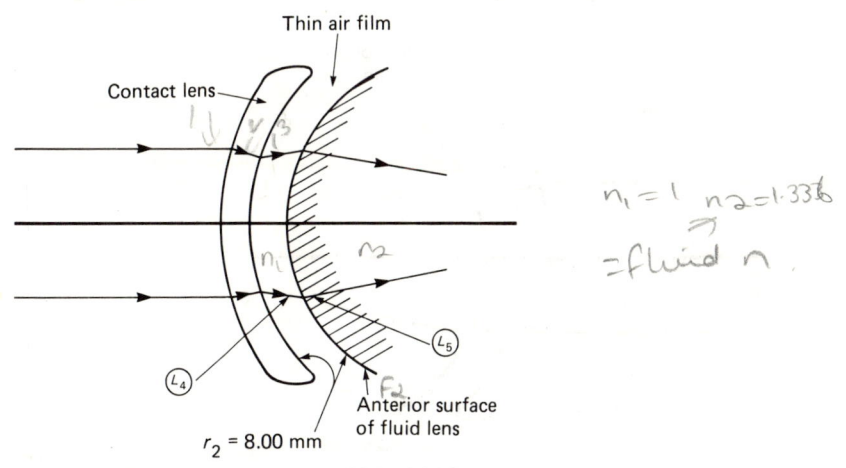

Figure 2.5. The lens to order for a BCOR of 8.00 mm.

The power of the fluid lens anterior surface is

$$\frac{336}{8} = +42.00 \text{ D}$$

Therefore the emergent vergence from the fluid lens anterior surface is

$$L_5 = +42.00 - 1.50 = +40.50 \text{ D}$$

We can therefore conclude that, if the emergent vergence from the anterior surface of the fluid lens is $+40.50$ D, then the lens will correct the refractive error.

2.5.1 The lens to be ordered

When the BCOR is changed this alters the power of the anterior surface of the fluid lens. However, all components posterior to this surface remain unchanged when the new BCOR is substituted. Therefore we can conclude that, if the emergent vergence from the anterior surface of the fluid lens is held at $+40.50$ D, then the new lens will still correct the refractive error.

In *Figure 2.6*, L_5 must be $+40.50$ D if this lens is still to correct the refractive error. The power of the fluid lens anterior surface is

$$\frac{336}{8.25} = +40.73 \text{ D}$$

∴ Vergence $L_4 = +40.50 - 40.73 = -0.23$ D

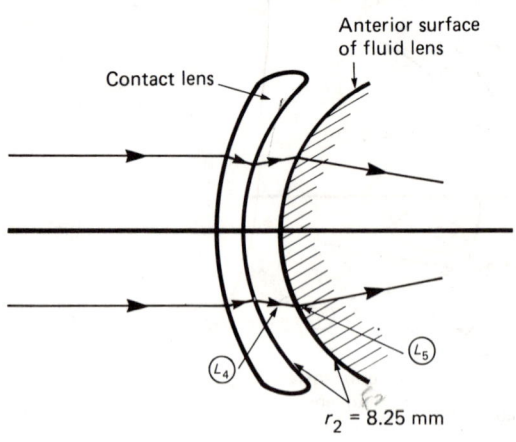

Figure 2.6. The lens to order for a BCOR of 8.25 mm. L_5 must be $+40.50$ D.

Since the air film is thin this is both the incident vergence on the fluid lens anterior surface and the emergent vergence from the back surface of the contact lens in air.

$$\therefore L_4 = -0.23 \, D = \text{BVP of contact lens in air}$$

N.B. We have calculated that a BCOR change of 0.25 mm must be accompanied by a power change of approximately 1.25 D. Thus a change of 0.05 mm in the BCOR must be accompanied by a fluid lens power change of 0.25 D. This approximate rule is well worth remembering since it not only allows deduction of the power to order but it tells the contact lens fitter whether the lens is steep, aligned or flat. If, for example, a 2.00 D myope was fitted with a contact lens and the over-refraction indicated that a BVP of −2.50 D was required, then this suggests that the fluid lens power is +0.50 D. If we use the approximate rule above we deduce that the contact lens is fitting 0.1 mm steep. The rule applies to scleral and corneal lenses, both hard (PMMA) and gas permeable (GPH), since the contact lens refractive index does not enter into the equation. However, it cannot be applied to soft lenses since they tend to take up the curvature of the central cornea on which they rest. Thus the power of the fluid lens is unpredictable but is likely to be approximately afocal and to remain largely unaltered by changes in the contact lens specification.

2.6 Contact lens over-refraction using a lens with an inappropriate BVP

If the over-refraction is performed using a contact lens which has a BVP considerably different from that required for correction of the ametropia, then errors may arise as illustrated below.

A scleral lens with a BVP of −12.00 D, central thickness 0.8 mm, a BCOR of 8.75 mm and a front central optic radius (FCOR) of 11.40 mm is used for an over-refraction. The end point of the over-refraction is reached when a +8.00 DS is interposed at a vertex distance of 12 mm from the contact lens. What BVP should be requested when the lens with a BCOR of 8.75 mm is ordered?

2.6.1 Approximate calculation in clinical practice

We would calculate the effective power of the +8.00 DS at the contact lens as follows:

38 The contact lens

	Vergence (D)		Distance (mm)
F_s	$= +8.00$	$\dfrac{1000}{8}$	$\rightarrow 125$
Effective power	$= +8.85 \leftarrow$	$\dfrac{1000}{113}$	$\dfrac{-12}{113} = \text{vertex distance}$

We then add this effective power to the BVP of the contact lens, giving

$$+8.85 - 12.00 = -3.15 \text{ D}$$

and this is the BVP that would be ordered.

2.6.2 Accurate calculation

In *Figure 2.7*,

front surface power of contact lens $F_1 = \dfrac{n-1}{r_1} = \dfrac{490}{11.4} = +43.00 \text{ D}$

back surface power of contact lens $F_2 = \dfrac{1-n}{r_2} = \dfrac{-490}{8.75} = -56.00 \text{ D}$

$t/n = \dfrac{0.8}{1.490} = 0.54 \text{ mm}$

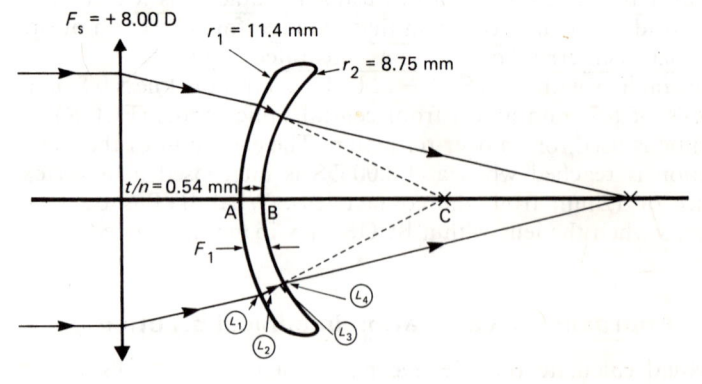

Figure 2.7. The over-refraction.

From *Figure 2.7*:

Vergence (D)	Distance (mm)

$L_1 = +8.85$

$F_1 = +43.00$

$L_2 = +51.85 \xrightarrow{\dfrac{1000}{51.85}} 19.29 = AC$

$\underline{-0.54 = t/n}$

$L_3 = +53.33 \xleftarrow{\dfrac{1000}{18.75}} 18.75$

$F_2 = -56.00$

$L_4 = -2.67\,D$ = accurate BVP in air

The clinical estimation of BVP was $-3.15\,D$ which is 0.48 D too negative.

This error arises from the fact that the spectacle lens used in the over-refraction is of high power and the contact lens is a thick lens with powerful surfaces. In the example illustrated above we have a high plus spectacle lens at a finite vertex distance which serves to magnify the retinal image. When the contact lens returns with the correct BVP, much of this magnification is lost and the visual acuity may not be as good as that found at the time of the over-refraction.

2.7 Modifying an existing lens

It is not uncommon in scleral lens fitting to change the BCOR of a lens by modifying the lens worn by the patient. A modified BCOR not only changes the power of the anterior surface of the fluid lens but also alters the BVP of the contact lens.

The following example illustrates these changes.

A contact lens of BCOR 8.25 mm, BVP $-3.00\,D$ and central thickness 0.6 mm corrects the ametropia but the optic must be reground to a BCOR of 8.75 mm. What is the new front surface radius required if the lens is still to correct the eye? What is the front vertex power of this modified lens? Assume that the contact lens and fluid lens centre thicknesses do not change.

2.7.1 Before modification

In *Figure 2.8(a)*

vergence incident on the anterior surface of the fluid lens = -3.00 D

power of the anterior surface of the fluid lens = $\dfrac{336}{8.25} = +40.73$ D

∴ Emergent vergence from the anterior surface of the fluid lens = $+40.73 - 3.00$

$= +37.73$ D

This must remain unchanged after modification.

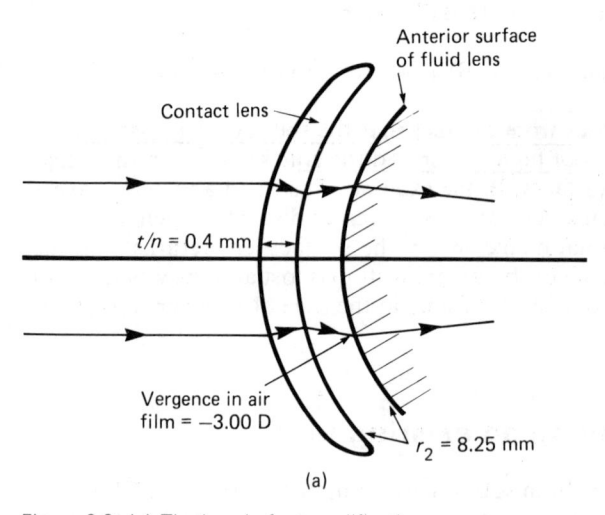

Figure 2.8. (a) The lens before modification.

2.7.2 After modification

Figure 2.8(b) shows the lens after modification. If this lens is still to correct the refractive error, then vergence L_5 must be $+37.73$ D. We can therefore use the step along method to calculate r_1.

Modifying an existing lens 41

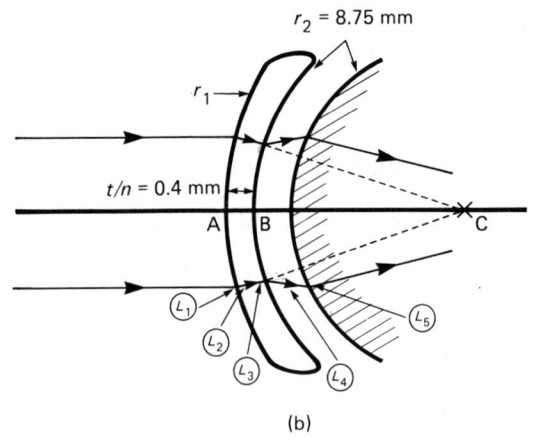

Figure 2.8. (b) The lens after modification. L_5 must be +37.73 D.

Power of anterior surface of fluid lens $= \dfrac{336}{8.75} = +38.40$ D

Power of back surface of contact lens $F_2 = \dfrac{-490}{8.75} = -56.00$ D

Reduced thickness $t/n = \dfrac{0.6}{1.490} = 0.4$ mm for the contact lens

| | Vergence (D) | Distance (mm) |

L_5 must be   +37.73

Power of anterior
surface of fluid lens = +38.40

$\therefore L_4 = -0.67 =$ BVP of contact lens in air
$F_2 = -56.00$

$\therefore L_3 = +55.33 \xrightarrow{\dfrac{1000}{55.33}} 18.07 = BC$

$\underline{0.4} = t/n$

$L_2 = +54.14 \xleftarrow{\dfrac{1000}{18.47}} 18.47 = AC$

$L_1 = \underline{00.00}$

Front surface
power $F_1 = +54.14$ ✓

42 The contact lens

$$r_1 = \frac{n-1}{F_1} = \frac{490}{54.14} = 9.05 \text{ mm}$$

must consider light as if entering from the back. So just turn diagram round.

2.7.3 Front vertex power (FVP)

Again if we work through the system illustrated in *Figure 2.9* using the step along method we can calculate the front vertex power.

	Vergence (D)		Distance (mm)
L_1 =	0.00		
F_2 =	-56.00		
L_2 =	-56.00 $\xrightarrow{\dfrac{1000}{-56}}$		$-17.86 = AB$
			$-0.4 = t/n$
L_3 =	-54.76 $\xleftarrow{\dfrac{1000}{-18.26}}$		$-18.26 = AC$
F_1 =	$+54.14$		
∴ L_4 =	-0.62		

∴ Front vertex power (FVP) = -0.62 D

There is a program in Chapter 7 which calculates FVP.
In the above example we assumed no change in the contact lens or fluid lens central thickness. Therefore a second example will be given to illustrate how the problem is treated when these thicknesses change along with a change of BCOR.
A scleral contact lens has a BCOR of 8.25 mm, a BVP of -3.00 D and central thickness of 0.6 mm. This corrects the ametropia but slight apical touch persuades the practitioner to regrind the optic to a BCOR of 8.00 mm. This reduces the contact lens thickness to 0.5 mm and increases the fluid lens thickness from zero to 0.1 mm. What is the new BVP required if the system is still to correct the

Modifying an existing lens 43

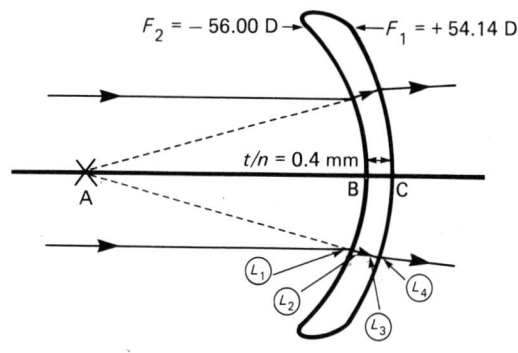

$F_2 = -56.00$ D $F_1 = +54.14$ D

$t/n = 0.4$ mm

Figure 2.9. Front vertex power. L_4 is the FVP.

ametropia? What front surface radius is required for the modified lens?

2.7.4 Before modification

The result is as in the previous example, i.e. the emergent vergence from the anterior surface of the fluid lens is $+37.73$ D. Since the fluid lens before modification has no thickness, this must also be the incident vergence on the posterior surface of the fluid lens. We conclude that this vergence must be maintained on this posterior surface.

2.7.5 After modification

After modification the contact lens/fluid lens system is as illustrated in *Figure 2.10*.

$r_2 = 8.00$ mm

Contact lens

Fluid lens

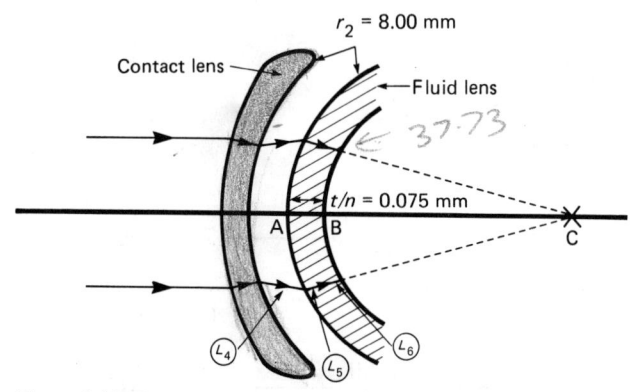

37.73

$t/n = 0.075$ mm

Figure 2.10. The system after modification. L_6 must be $+37.73$ D.

Power of anterior surface of fluid lens $= \dfrac{n-1}{r_2} = \dfrac{336}{8} = +42.00$ D

Reduced thickness of fluid lens $= t/n = \dfrac{0.1}{1.336} = 0.075$ mm

	Vergence (D)		Distance (mm)
L_6 must be	$+37.73$ —— $\dfrac{1000}{37.73}$ —→	$26.50 = $ BC
			$0.075 = t/n$
$L_5 =$	$+37.63$ ←—— $\dfrac{1000}{26.575}$ ——	$26.575 = $ AC

Power of anterior surface of fluid lens
$\quad = \quad +42.00$

$\therefore L_4 = \quad -4.37 = $ BVP of contact lens in air

In *Figure 2.11* the power of the back surface of the contact lens is

$$F_2 = \dfrac{1-n}{r_2} = \dfrac{-490}{8} = -61.25 \text{ D}$$

Reduced thickness of contact lens $= t/n = \dfrac{0.5}{1.490} = 0.34$ mm

	Vergence (D)		Distance (mm)
L_4 must be	-4.37		
F_2	$= -61.25$		
$\therefore L_3$	$= +56.88$ —— $\dfrac{1000}{56.88}$ —→	$17.58 = $ BC
			$0.34 = t/n$
L_2	$= +55.80$ ←—— $\dfrac{1000}{17.92}$ ——	$17.92 = $ AC

Modifying an existing lens 45

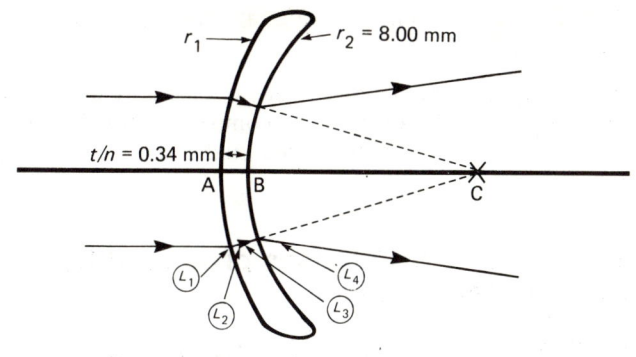

[Figure: diagram showing modified contact lens with r_1, $r_2 = 8.00$ mm, $t/n = 0.34$ mm, points A, B, C, and lens vergences L_1, L_2, L_3, L_4]

Figure 2.11. The modified contact lens. L_4 must be -4.37 D.

$$L_1 = \underline{\quad 00.00 \quad}$$

$\therefore F_1 = +55.80 =$ power of the front surface of the contact lens

$$r_1 = \frac{n-1}{F_1} = \frac{490}{55.8} = 8.78 \text{ mm}$$

Thus the only difference between the first and second example of lens modification is that in the first example we maintained the vergence at the anterior fluid surface but in the second a fluid lens thickness change results in the anterior surface changing position, and so we must maintain the vergence of light at the fluid lens posterior surface.

2.7.6 Approximate rules

There are two approximate rules that can be used clinically when modifying scleral lenses.

(1) For each reduction of 0.05 mm in BCOR, $+0.12$ D must be added to the altered BVP of the contact lens in order to maintain correction by the contact lens/fluid lens system.

(2) A reduction of the contact lens central thickness of 0.1 mm must be accompanied by a $+0.25$ D change in power. However, if this also increases the fluid lens central thickness by 0.1 mm then this will require a further power modification of

−0.12 D. Thus in these circumstances the total power modification is +0.12 D.

It may therefore be advisable to order scleral lenses about 0.50 D more positive than the refraction result to compensate for the optic grind outs (usually about 0.2 mm total) required due to the settling of the contact lens.

2.8 The BVP of scleral lenses produced by the impression technique

One of the advantages of the impression technique is that the practitioner does not require expensive fitting sets that will be used on a small number of patients during his or her fitting career. The suggestion therefore that a fenestrated lens for optic measurement (FLOM) be used as part of a contact lens over-refraction is self-defeating. The impression technique produces a contact lens which matches the scleral topography. The optic specification is usually ordered by asking for an optic radius 0.2–0.5 mm flatter than the flattest keratometry reading and specifying a central clearance from the cast. The central clearance for a first impression is usually 0.2 mm, which should result in a contact lens apical clearance of about 0.1 mm. Let us suppose that the keratometry reading is 7.60 mm spherical and that the eye is 3.00 D myopic. The power of the fluid lens can be deduced using the approximate rule that a 0.1 mm radius change produces 0.50 D power change in the fluid lens. In this example, suppose we used a back optic radius of 7.8 mm (0.2 mm flatter than the keratometry reading); then the fluid lens power is −1.00 D. The contact lens BVP ordered must therefore be −2.00 to correct this 3.00 D myopic eye. It must be emphasized that this is an approximation which also ignores the effect of the fluid lens thickness. However, the BVP of the contact lens at worst will only need minor modification.

A more accurate BVP can be deduced just as easily using Heine's scale to deduce the surface powers of the fluid lens and adding them algebraically to give the fluid lens power. This still leaves the influence of the fluid lens thickness unaccounted for. However, if the ideal apical clearance of about 0.1 mm is achieved in the fitting, this will only add approximately +0.12 D to the power of the fluid lens.

2.9 Heine's scale

In the early days of scleral contact lens fitting, a technique was used by Heine which involved correcting the ametropia with afocal contact lenses. This inevitably means that the fluid lens is used to correct the refractive error. We can deduce the power of the fluid lens in air using the equation

$$F = \frac{n-1}{r}$$

This allows us to calculate the surface powers of the fluid lens, and these can be simply added together to give total lens power if we assume that the fluid lens is thin. The back surface of the fluid lens is determined by the corneal curvature and this can be measured using a keratometer. Let us suppose that a 2.00 D myope has a keratometry reading of 7.4 mm.

Power of posterior surface of fluid lens
$$= \frac{1-n}{r} = \frac{-336}{7.4} = -45.41 \text{ D}$$

The fluid lens is assumed to be thin and must have a BVP of −2.00 D to correct the myopia.

∴ Power of anterior surface of fluid lens = +43.41 D

∴ Radius of anterior surface of fluid lens
$$= \frac{n-1}{F} = \frac{336}{43.41} = 7.74 \text{ mm}$$

In a clinical situation all that is needed is a table or scale which converts power to radius assuming a refractive index of 1.336. *Figure 2.12* shows a section of Heine's scale. The scale is used to convert radii to surface powers or surface powers to radii.

The scale was originally calibrated for a refractive index of 1.332 and later modified to 1.336 by Bennett. The reader can construct such a scale or table easily by using the equation $F = (n-1)/r$ in

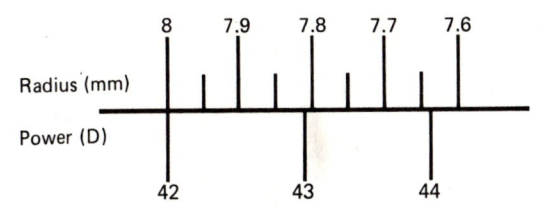

Figure 2.12. A small section of Heine's scale.

radius steps of 0.05 mm. There is a computer program in Chapter 7 which makes the conversion for a medium of any refractive index.

Note that in the above example, if we applied the approximation that 0.1 mm radius difference produces a 0.50 D power change in the fluid lens, we would order a contact lens with BCOR of 7.4 mm (the keratometry reading) plus 0.4 mm (the flattening required for a −2.00 D fluid lens) which gives a total of 7.8 mm, and this actually results in the fluid lens BVP being −2.33 D.

2.9.1 Thickness

For average radii, each 0.1 mm increase in fluid lens thickness adds +0.12 D to the effective power of the system. Therefore, if the fluid lens is thick, the BCOR of the contact lens (r_2) should be increased an appropriate amount to adjust the fluid lens power.

2.10 Edge and centre thickness

The deduction of either the centre or the edge thickness of a contact lens when the other contact lens surface parameters are known revolves around the use of the sag equation.

2.10.1 The sag equation

Figure 2.13 has the appearance of a bow and arrow with the bow pulled taut prior to firing. The vertical line in the diagram is the arrow and dimension *s* is called the sag, which is derived from the latin word *sagitta* meaning arrow. The size of *s* will be determined by the radius of curvature of the curved surface *r* and the length of the chord 2*y*.

In *Figure 2.13*, by Pythagoras' theorem,

$$r^2 = y^2 + (r-s)^2$$

$$\therefore (r-s)^2 = r^2 - y^2$$

$$r - s = \sqrt{r^2 - y^2}$$

$$s = r - \sqrt{r^2 - y^2}$$

A typical example is illustrated below.

Edge and centre thickness 49

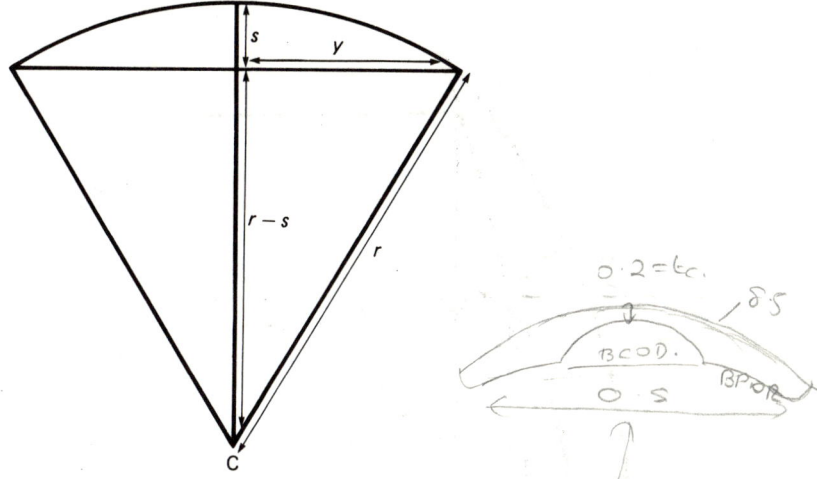

Figure 2.13. The sag of a spherical surface. s is the sag; y is the semi-diameter; r is the radius of curvature of the surface; C is the centre of curvature.

What is the axial edge thickness 4.25 mm from the centre of the following contact lens:

C2 7.60;6.50/10.50;10.00

if the front surface radius is 8.50 mm and the lens centre thickness is 0.2 mm?

The only real problem with this type of example is drawing the diagram correctly. *Figure 2.14* illustrates the contact lens cross section where it can readily be seen that the axial edge thickness (t_e) equals the total sag minus the sag of the front surface. The total sag is easily seen to be $s_1 + s_2 - s_3 + t_c$. All that remains therefore is to calculate sags s_1, s_2, s_3 and the front surface sag. On multicurve lenses the relationship can be extended as follows: if the next curve has sags of s_4 for its outer diameter and s_5 for its inner diameter, then we obtain the equation

total sag $= s_1 + s_2 - s_3 + s_4 - s_5 + t_c$

For s_1

$s_1 = 7.60 - \sqrt{7.60^2 - 3.25^2}$

$= 7.60 - 6.87$

$= 0.73$ mm

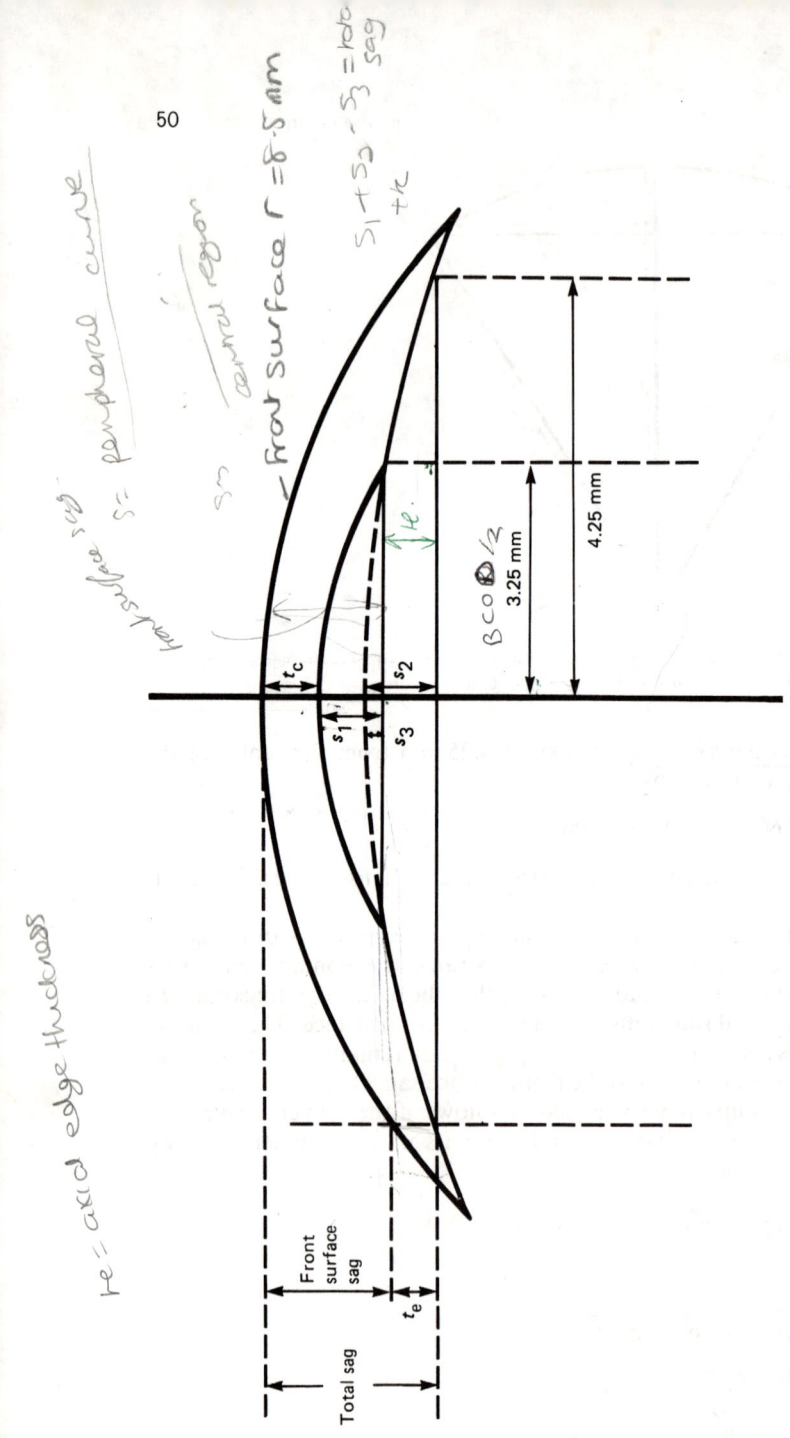

Figure 2.14. The sags of the contact lens back surface. t_c is the centre thickness. t_e is the axial edge thickness.

For s_2

$s_2 = 10.50 - \sqrt{10.50^2 - 4.25^2}$

$= 10.50 - 9.60$

$= 0.9$ mm

For s_3

$s_3 = 10.50 - \sqrt{10.50^2 - 3.25^2}$

$= 10.50 - 9.98$

$= 0.52$ mm

$\therefore s_1 + s_2 - s_3 + t_c = 1.31$ mm $=$ total sag

Front surface sag

$s = 8.50 - \sqrt{8.50^2 - 4.25^2}$

$= 8.50 - 7.36$

$= 1.14$ mm

Axial edge thickness $=$ total sag $-$ sag of front surface

$= 1.31 - 1.14$

$= 0.17$ mm

There is a computer program in Chapter 7 which will calculate axial edge thickness for C2, C3 and C4 lenses.

2.11 Edge lift

Axial edge lift is treated in much the same way as edge and centre thickness problems, as is shown in the following example.
 Calculate the axial edge lift of the corneal lens

 C3 7.80:7.00/8.80:8.00/11.00:8.60

In *Figure 2.15* we can see that the axial edge lift is equal to s_6 minus the primary sag, and

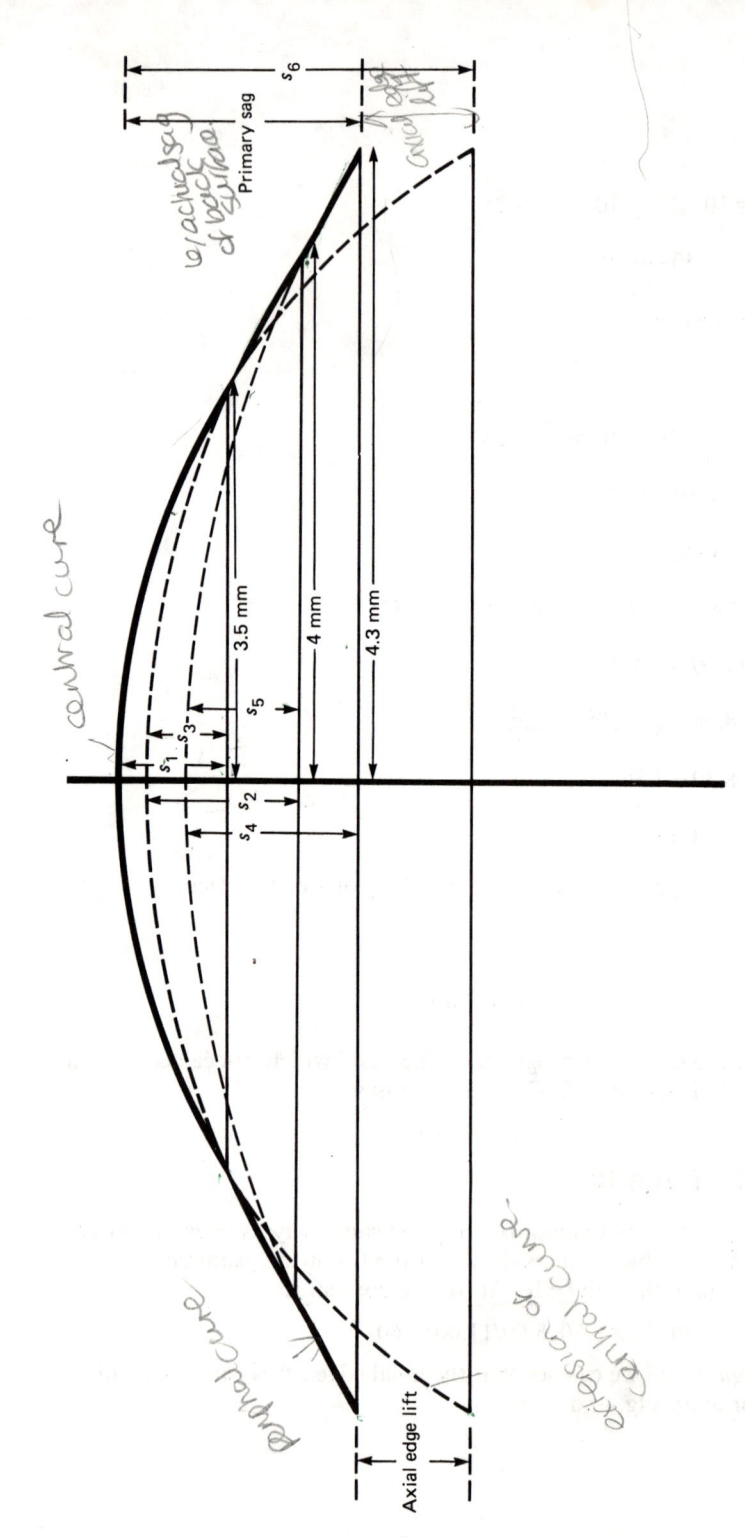

Figure 2.15. Axial edge lift. The values 3.5, 4, and 4.3 are the semi-diameters of the lens.

Edge lift 53

primary sag = $s_1 + s_2 - s_3 + s_4 - s_5$

For s_1

$s_1 = 7.80 - \sqrt{7.80^2 - 3.5^2}$

= 0.83 mm

For s_2

$s_2 = 8.80 - \sqrt{8.80^2 - 4^2}$

= 0.96 mm

For s_3

$s_3 = 8.80 - \sqrt{8.80^2 - 3.5^2}$

= 0.73 mm

For s_4

$s_4 = 11.00 - \sqrt{11.00^2 - 4.3^2}$

= 0.88 mm

For s_5

$s_5 = 11.00 - \sqrt{11.00^2 - 4^2}$

= 0.75 mm

For s_6

$s_6 = 7.80 - \sqrt{7.80^2 - 4.3^2}$

= 1.29 mm

Primary sag = 1.19 mm — from above formula

Axial edge lift = s_6 − primary sag

= 1.29 − 1.19

= 0.1 mm

problems of axial edge & edge liftare simular

54 The contact lens

There is a computer program in Chapter 7 that calculates the axial and radial edge lift of C2, C3 and C4 lenses. There is also a program which calculates the back surface peripheral radii required to give a specified edge lift for C2, C3 and C4 lenses. A C4 lens has a primary sag of $s_1 + s_2 - s_3 + s_4 - s_5 + s_6 - s_7$. The equation used to derive radial edge lift is given below.

In practice an instrument similar to the sag-measuring devices (derived from the lens measure) currently used for deducing the radius of curvature of soft lenses is required for measurement of edge lift. Stone (1975) has suggested an adaptation of the radiuscope (optical spherometer) for measuring the lens sag. This involves the use of a supporting cylindrical pillar of accurately known diameter $2y$ (see *Figure 2.16*). The radiuscope is focussed on the flat top of the pillar. The contact lens is placed on the top of the pillar and the radiuscope is refocussed on to the convex anterior lens surface. The primary sag will be the movement of the radiuscope between these two positions minus the lens centre thickness.

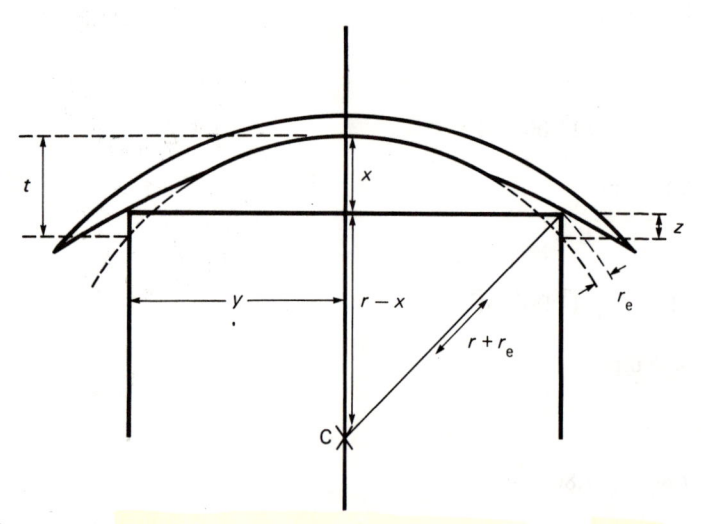

Figure 2.16. Measurement of x to deduce the radial edge lift r_e and the axial lift z. C is the centre of curvature of the back central optic of radius r.

From Pythagoras' theorem in *Figure 2.16*

$$(r + r_e)^2 = (r - x)^2 + y^2$$

where r is the BCOR, r_e is the radial edge lift, and x is the primary sag measured on the cylindrical supporting pillar of semi-diameter y.

Therefore the radial edge lift is

$$r_e = \sqrt{(r-x)^2 + y^2} - r$$

The notion of using radial edge lift was suggested by Hodd (1966). *Figure 2.16* also illustrates that the axial edge lift z is the sag of the central curve t over a diameter $2y$ minus the primary sag measured by the radiuscope:

Axial edge lift $z = t - x$

t can be easily calculated if the BCOR is measured and y is known. The above technique can also be used for checking the edge lift of offset and aspheric back surface lenses.

The relationship between radial edge lift and axial edge lift is not exactly constant; however, the ratio varies little over typical contact lens parameter variation. The radial-to-axial ratio is around 0.8 for an axial edge lift of 0.175 mm. A constant axial edge lift gives more radial lift on flat lenses; however, the increase in radial lift with increase in BCOR typically amounts to something around 0.016 mm from the flattest to the steepest lens.

One final point that should be made on the topic of edge lift is that, as the BCOR of a lens is increased, the degree of flattening of the peripheral curve or curves must be increased to maintain a particular edge lift; i.e. if, say, a bicurve lens with BCOR of 7.5 mm provided the required edge lift when the BPOR equals the BCOR plus 1 mm, a flatter lens of, say, BCOR 8.2 mm will require a BPOR greater than the BCOR plus 1 mm in order to achieve the same edge lift.

2.12 Aspheric contact lens surfaces

In the contact lens world the term 'aspheric surface' can be taken to mean a conicoid-like surface. The conicoid arises from a curve which is derived by taking a section through a cone. These curves are determined by the orientation of the section. If the section is parallel to the base of the cone then the curve is circular, which will produce a spherical surface. This must obviously be the one curve that is excluded from this classification. As the section is made more oblique to the base of the cone, the curve becomes increasingly elliptical until it reaches a parabolic form where it then changes to a hyperbola. These curves give rise to surfaces which are spherical, ellipsoidal, paraboloidal and hyperboloidal, and the degree of flattening with eccentricity will depend upon the precise characteristics of the surface. A hyperboloidal surface, for instance, produces a peripheral flattening that may well be excessive for contact lens use, whereas a sphere produces no peripheral flattening at all. Bennett (1968) suggested using the concept of a z value as a method of specifying the departure of a surface from that of a spherical surface which has the same radius of curvature at the vertex. The z value has since been described as the axial edge lift and is illustrated in *Figure 2.17*. N.B. At any point on a conicoid except the vertex, the curvature changes in different meridians.

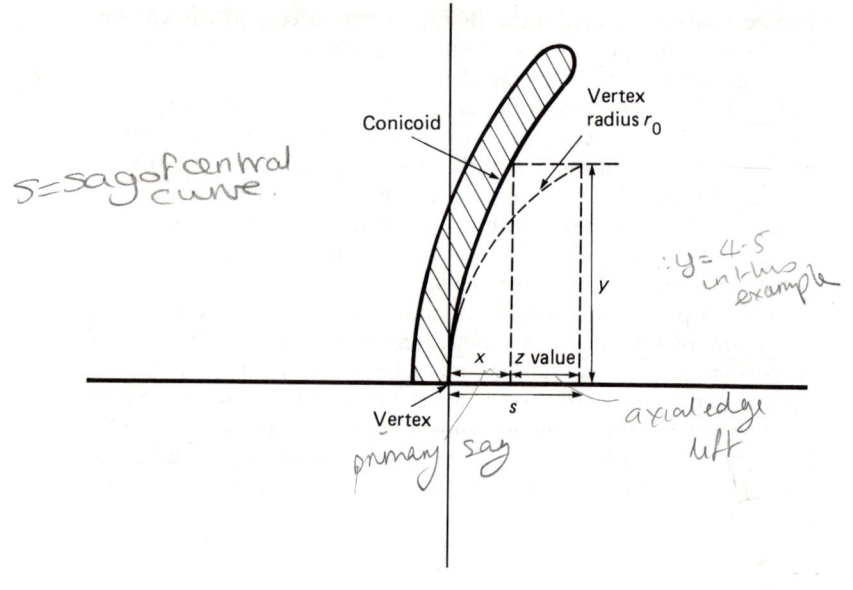

Figure 2.17. Determination of the conicoid required to give a specific z value.

Suppose we required a lens with a central vertex radius r_0 of 7.60 mm and an overall size $2y$ of 9.00 mm with an axial edge lift z of 0.1 mm. In *Figure 2.17* we can determine the sag (s) of the spherical surface of radius r_0. If we then subtract the z value from this we acquire the primary sag x. We must then use the conic section equation

$$p = \frac{2r_0 x - y^2}{x^2}$$

in order to deduce p which defines the conic section for vertex radius r_0.

Aspheric contact lens surfaces 57

For the sphere

$$s = r_0 - \sqrt{r_0^2 - y^2}$$
$$= 7.6 - \sqrt{7.6^2 - 4.5^2}$$
$$s = 1.48 \text{ mm}$$

From *Figure 2.17*

$$x = s - z$$
$$= 1.48 - 0.1$$
$$x = 1.38 \text{ mm}$$

For the conicoid

$$p = \frac{2r_0 x - y^2}{x^2}$$
$$= \frac{2 \times 7.6 \times 1.38 - 4.5^2}{1.38^2}$$

$$p = 0.38$$

p describes the curve, since p is 1 for a sphere; p lies between zero and +1 for an ellipsoid (an oblate ellipsoid); p is zero for a paraboloid; and p is negative for a hyperboloid. Thus in the above example the conicoid required is an oblate (flattening) ellipsoid where $p = 0.38$.

If we needed to check this surface then we must refer again to the conic section equation

$$p = \frac{2r_0 x - y^2}{x^2}$$

The value of p depends on r_0, y and x.

If the vertex radius r_0 is found to be correct and the semi-diameter y has been fixed, then a measurement of x can be used to check the manufacturer's precision. The checking can be performed using a modified radiuscope as outlined in Section 2.11. We need to measure the value of x over a specific aperture $2y$. The best accuracy can be achieved with a large aperture, but from a practical point of view this would have to be limited to about 8 mm to eliminate inaccuracies arising from the edge taper. Therefore, in order to check our lens, we must measure the value x and compare this with the value deduced from the relationship $x = s - z = 1.38$ mm. The radial edge lift can be determined using

$$r_e = \sqrt{(r_0 - x)^2 + y^2} - r_0$$

2.12.1 Calculating x

To calculate x we can use the expression

$$x = (r_0/p) - \sqrt{(r_0/p)^2 - y^2/p}$$

In the case of a sphere, where $p = 1$, the equation is simplified to $x = r_0 - \sqrt{r_0^2 - y^2}$ which is the familiar sag equation for a spherical surface. For a parabola, where $p = 0$, the conic section equation reduces to

$$y^2 = 2r_0 x$$

hardly ever encounter a parabola.

$$\therefore x = \frac{y^2}{2r_0}$$

Alternatively, if the vertex radius is known, we can calculate x from the simple relationship

$$x = s - z$$

for any given edge lift at any particular diameter.

There is a computer program in Chapter 7 which calculates the values x and p for aspheric surfaces.

Numerical substitution in the above equations indicates that the z value decreases with increase in vertex radius for an ellipsoid or paraboloid. The only other term that you may encounter is the surface eccentricity e. The relationship between p and e is

$$p = 1 - e^2$$

2.13 Offset or continuous bicurve lenses

It is not an easy matter to produce a conicoid surface. The surface production can be made easier by generating a surface which approximates to the conicoid. This can be achieved as illustrated in *Figure 2.18*.

The central region of the lens is spherical with a suitable BCOR r_1 and BCOD (back central optic diameter) y_1. The peripheral section has a BPOR r_2 with the centre of curvature C_2 lying offset from the axis AC_1. Since these two curves have a common normal at B there will be no visible transition as occurs in a conventional bicurve design. The centre of curvature C_2 is offset to the opposite side of the axis, and this has been termed by Ruben (1966) a contralateral offset bicurve. The peripheral surface which results from this type of construction is an eccentric zone of a barrel toric. The z value is

Offset or continuous bicurve lenses

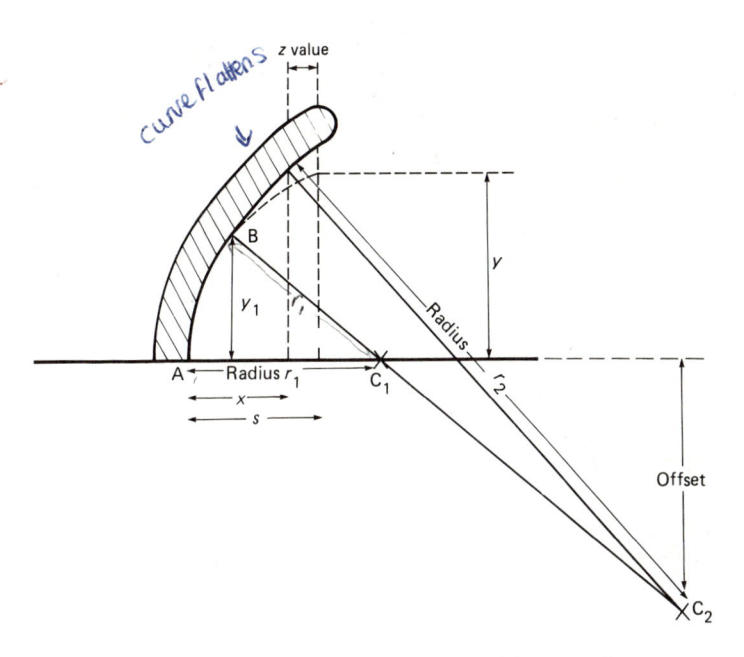

Figure 2.18. The contralateral offset or continuous bicurve surface.

determined by the peripheral radius and the offset. Inspection of *Figure 2.18* should lead to the conclusion that these are interdependent since C_2 must always lie on the line $B\,C_1\,C_2$.

In order to check that the axial edge lift is as requested, we can resort to a similar inspection to that for the conicoid. In *Figure 2.18* we can see that a measurement of the primary sag of the lens over an aperture $2y$ (which must be larger than the BCOD) provides us with the value x. s can be calculated from the sag equation

$$s = r_1 - \sqrt{r_1^2 - y^2}$$

and the z value deduced from the relationship

z value $= s - x$

Once again the radial edge lift can be found using

$$r_e = \sqrt{(r-x)^2 + y^2} - r$$

Alternatively a radius could be given for the peripheral curve and a

60 The contact lens

calculation of the z value would be required in order to compare this with the result acquired by measurement using the method just described.

An example will be used for illustration.

A contralateral offset bicurve lens is made to the following specification: BCOR 7.60 mm; BCOD 6.00 mm; BPOR 12 mm; OS 9.50 mm. What is the axial edge lift at a diameter of 9.00 mm?

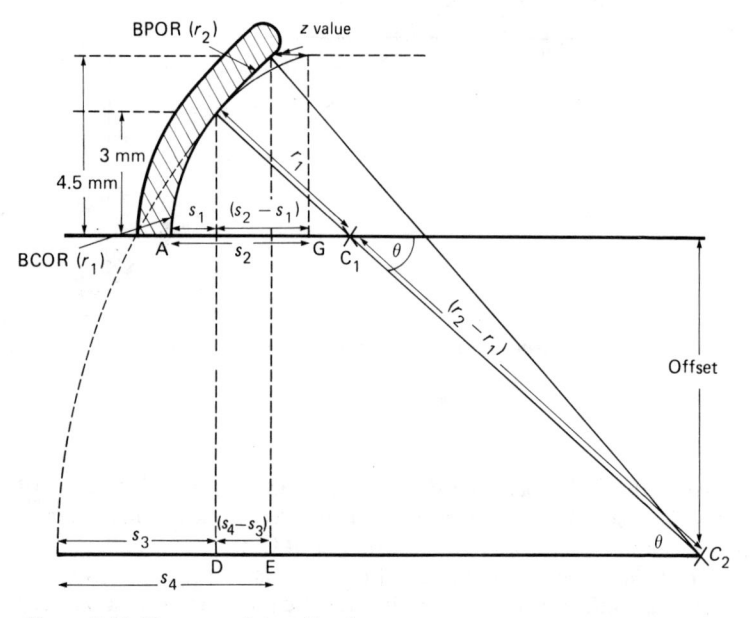

Figure 2.19. The sags of the offset lens.

From *Figure 2.19* we can see that

z value $= (s_2 - s_1) - (s_4 - s_3)$

$s_1 = 7.60 - \sqrt{7.60^2 - 3^2} = 0.617$ mm

$s_2 = 7.60 - \sqrt{7.60^2 - 4.5^2} = 1.475$ mm

$s_2 - s_1 = 0.858$ mm

For s_3 and s_4 we must first calculate the semi-diameters which must include the offset. From *Figure 2.19*

$$\sin\theta = \frac{\frac{1}{2}\text{BCOD}}{\text{BCOR}} = \frac{3.00}{7.60} = 0.3947$$

but

$$\sin\theta = \frac{\text{offset}}{r_2 - r_1}$$

$$\therefore \text{Offset} = (r_2 - r_1)\sin\theta = 1.737 \text{ mm}$$

We can now calculate s_3 and s_4:

$$s_3 = 12 - \sqrt{12^2 - 4.737^2} = 0.975 \text{ mm}$$

$$s_4 = 12 - \sqrt{12^2 - 6.237^2} = 1.748 \text{ mm}$$

$$s_4 - s_3 = 0.773 \text{ mm}$$

z value = (s₂−s₁) − (s₄−s₃)

z value $= 0.858 - 0.773$

z value $= 0.085$ mm   *true for aspherical lenses*

The investigation of a range of surface radii reveals that, if we assume that the cornea is ellipsoidal or paraboloidal in form, then flatter corneas display less axial edge lift. If we wish to maintain edge lift in a contact lens fitting set then the peripheral curves of flatter lenses must possess a greater degree of flattening than that which occurs in the steeper lenses. Stone (1975) and Rabbetts (1976) have recommended the concept of constant edge lift for corneal fitting sets; however, they point out that edge lift refers to a measurement from the central spherical curve of the contact lens and that this is therefore not a clearance from the cornea. It may seem more rational to recommend a constant edge clearance from the cornea but this implies a detailed knowledge of an individual cornea which makes the concept somewhat theoretical at the moment. However, accepting that flatter corneas display less axial edge lift than steep corneas, perhaps the recommendation of constant edge lift fitting sets requires some reappraisal and may help to explain why fitting sets which maintain a fixed difference between BCOR and BPOR have been successful in the past.

corneal axial edge lifts- not as extractive as people suggest.

2.14 Prismatic effects with contact lenses

Prismatic effects in the case of a corneal contact lens fitted on or near alignment will be small due to the relatively small movement of the contact lens. The prism at the pupil centre can be deduced using the equation

$P = Fc$

where P is the prism power in prism dioptres (Δ), F is the BVP of the contact lens in dioptres, and c is the decentration of the optical centre of the contact lens from the pupil centre in centimetres. The fluid lens undergoes no change in these circumstances since the back surface of the contact lens rotates about its own centre of curvature when the lens decentres.

A scleral lens, however, will rotate about the centre of curvature of the scleral portion upon decentration and this will displace the anterior surface of the fluid lens. The prism produced will therefore be due to both the contact lens decentration and the displacement of the anterior surface of the fluid lens.

Figure 2.20 illustrates a scleral lens that is riding low. The optical centre of the contact lens is decentred a mm from the visual axis. The centre of curvature of the anterior surface of the fluid lens is displaced from C_2 (its position if the lens were well centred) to C_2'.

The prism at the corneal vertex is due to:

(1) the decentration of the contact lens;
(2) the displacement of the anterior surface of the fluid lens.

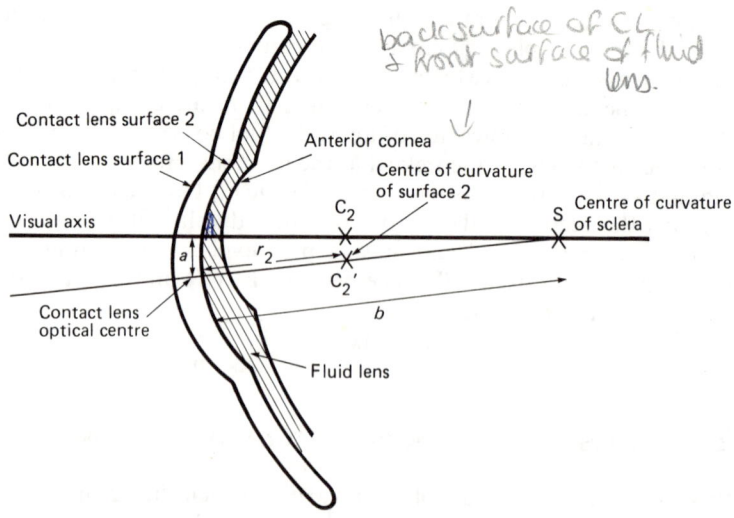

Figure 2.20. A low riding scleral contact lens.

Figure 2.20 illustrates that the fluid lens is producing a base-down prism, which can also be deduced from the fact that the visual axis passes through the upper region of the fluid lens anterior surface which obviously always has a positive power.

2.14.1 Prism due to the contact lens

If the contact lens has a BVP of F D in air and is decentred a mm then

$$\text{prism due to decentration} = \frac{aF}{10}$$

This will be base up for a negative lens, or base down for a positive when the lens rides low.

2.14.2 Prism due to the fluid lens anterior surface

Only the anterior surface of the fluid lens is changed by the lens decentration. We will therefore consider this surface only. A single refracting surface has no optical centre. The optical centre of a lens is the point which produces no deviation of light rays. The equivalent in a single refracting surface is the centre of curvature, in that any light ray directed to the centre of curvature will not be deviated as it crosses the surface. Therefore, if we can deduce the displacement of the centre of curvature from the visual axis and multiply this by the power of the surface, we will acquire the prism power due to the anterior surface displacement.

In *Figure 2.20*, by similar triangles

$$\frac{C_2 C_2'}{a} = \frac{b - r_2}{b} = 1 - \frac{r_2}{b}$$

$$\therefore C_2 C_2' = a\left(1 - \frac{r_2}{b}\right) \text{ mm}$$

The power of the anterior surface of the fluid lens is

$$F_L = \frac{336}{r_2}$$

$$\therefore \text{Prism power } \Delta = \frac{C_2 C_2' F_L}{10}$$

$$= \frac{a(1-r_2/b)(336/r_2)}{10}$$

$$= a\left(\frac{33.6}{r_2} - \frac{33.6}{b}\right) \text{ base down}$$

N.B. a, r_2 and b are all in millimetres.

2.14.3 Total prism

The total prism produced by decentration is obtained by adding together the prism due to the contact lens and the prism due to the fluid lens anterior surface.

2.15 Summary

- A 0.1 mm radius difference between the anterior cornea and posterior contact lens surface produces a fluid lens power of approximately 0.50 D. This is a most useful rule of thumb which can be used to advantage many times in clinical work.
- Avoid using a trial contact lens with a BVP that requires a high powered lens in the refractor head at the end point of the over-refraction.
- When modifying scleral lenses, each reduction of 0.05 mm in BCOR must be accompanied by a power change of +0.12 D to the BVP of the modified lens. A reduction of the contact lens central thickness of 0.1 mm must be accompanied by a +0.25 D change in lens power. However, if this also increases the fluid lens central thickness by 0.1 mm then this will require a further power modification of −0.12 D, making the total power change +0.12 D.
- Any calculation involving the first rule above can be made more precise by constructing a table based on the relationship

$$F = \frac{1.336 - 1}{r_2}$$

This is Heine's scale.

- The sag equation is

$$s = r - \sqrt{r^2 - y^2}$$

- The conic section equation is
$$p = \frac{2r_0 x - y^2}{x^2}$$
- The radial edge lift equation is
$$r_e = \sqrt{(r-x)^2 + y^2} - r$$
- For a constant axial edge lift, the peripheral radii will require relatively larger values on a flat lens.
- The axial edge lift decreases for an aspheric surface as the vertex radius is increased.
- The prismatic effect of a decentred contact lens will follow the Prentice rule
$$P = Fc$$

when the back surface of the contact lens rotates about its own centre of curvature. Where this is not the case the prismatic effect of the decentred anterior fluid lens surface must also be taken into account.

3 Measurement of the cornea

3.1 The keratometer

The keratometer is an ophthalmic instrument which utilizes a self-luminous object (the mire) to produce an image by reflection in the cornea. If we know the size and position of an object and the size and position of the image formed by reflection at the surface of a convex mirror, we can deduce the radius of curvature of that reflecting surface. Thus the keratometer is essentially a device for measuring image size.

3.2 The keratometer equation

In *Figure 3.1* we can see that a self-luminous target (the mire of a keratometer) can be used as an object which produces an image by reflection at the anterior surface of the cornea. This arrangement

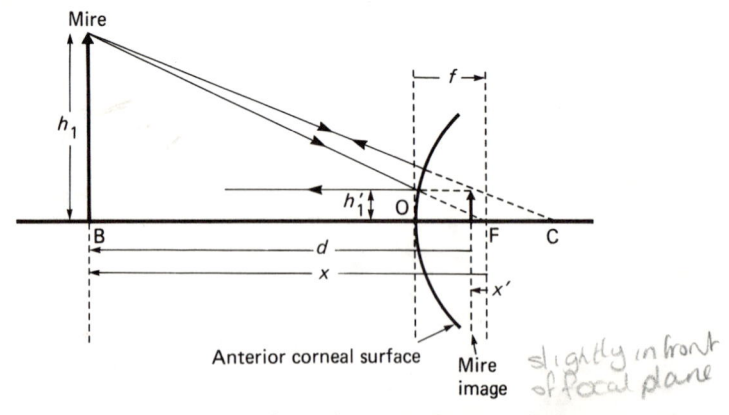

Figure 3.1. The formation of the mire image. The image is formed by reflection of light rays by the anterior corneal surface. This surface has a centre of curvature at C and a focal plane at F.

allows us to derive the radius of curvature of the cornea (r) as follows. Magnification can be defined as

$$\frac{\text{size of image}}{\text{size of object}} = \frac{h_1'}{h_1}$$

in *Figure 3.1*. By similar triangles

$$\frac{h_1'}{h_1} = \frac{\text{OF}}{\text{FB}} = -\frac{f}{x}$$

but for a convex mirror

$$f = \frac{r}{2}$$

$$\therefore \frac{h_1'}{h_1} = -\frac{r/2}{x} = -\frac{r}{2x}$$

$$\therefore r = -2\frac{h_1'}{h_1}x$$

If we were designing a keratometer we would need to decide on a value for the mire size h_1, and we would measure the mire image size h_1'. The only other value required to determine the radius of the anterior cornea is the distance x from the focal plane F to the mire B. If we knew the position of the focal plane we could deduce the corneal radius since $f = r/2$, and so it is obvious that we cannot know x unless we already know r. We must therefore make the approximation that x and d are equal, where d is the distance from the mire to the mire image. The equation now becomes

as x is from focal plane

$$r \approx -2\frac{h_1'}{h_1}d$$

The radius of curvature of the anterior cornea is acquired if we know the values h_1', h_1 and d. As already stated the mire size h_1 would be decided upon during the design of a particular instrument. Let us now look at how the values d and h_1' are deduced.

3.2.1 To deduce *d*

In *Figure 3.2* the keratometer position is adjusted until an image h_1'' is formed in the plane of the eyepiece crosswire. This fixes the image distance l' and must also fix the object distance l. If the mires are mounted on the instrument in the same plane as the objective then l

68 Measurement of the cornea

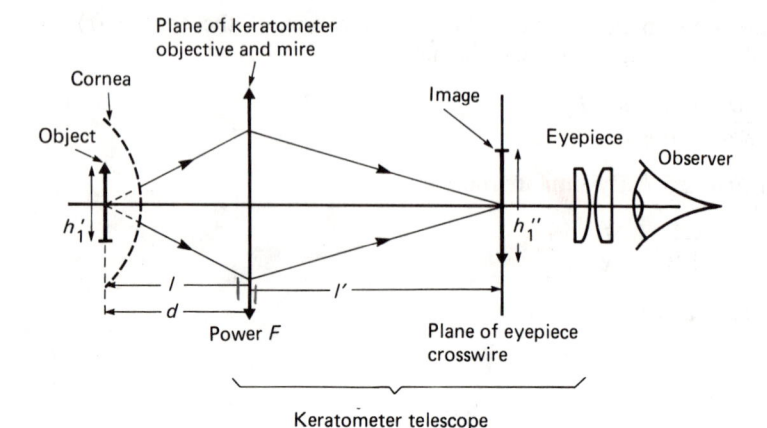

Figure 3.2. The mire image h_1' formed by the cornea becomes the object for the keratometer telescope which is positioned so that an image h_1'' is formed in the plane of the eyepiece crosswire. The distance from the telescope objective to the crosswire is the image distance l', which fixes a value for the object distance l. If the mire is mounted in the same plane as the objective then l equals d (the distance from the mire to the corneal image).

equals d since d in the keratometer equation is the distance between the mire and the corneal image h_1'.

In designing a keratometer we would select a value for the power of the objective lens and the distance between the objective and the crosswire, i.e. we would know the values for the lens power and the image distance and so deduction of the object distance is a simple matter of using the equation

$$\frac{1}{f} = \frac{1}{l'} - \frac{1}{l}$$

If the mires do not coincide with the objective it is simply a matter of adding or subtracting the distance between mire and objective to or from the value l in order to acquire d.

3.2.2 To deduce h_1'

Let us assume in *Figure 3.2* that h_1' and h_1'' represent the size of the object and image respectively for the telescope objective. Then we can use the relationship

$$\frac{\text{size of image}}{\text{size of object}} = \frac{\text{image distance}}{\text{object distance}}$$

which in *Figure 3.2* is

$$\frac{h_1''}{h_1'} = \frac{l'}{l}$$

$$\therefore h_1' = \frac{l}{l'} h_1''$$

Thus we can deduce h_1' if the other three values are known.

The values l and l' have already been decided upon during the design of the instrument as described above. We must therefore measure h_1'', the size of the image in the plane of the eyepiece crosswire. If we can measure this image size then we have everything required to substitute values in the keratometer equation to find the radius of curvature of the anterior surface of the cornea r.

keratometer – image size measuring device.
if image not in plane of crosswire, then l' will be wrong.

3.3 Doubling *: get inaccurate result.*

Head and eye movements on the part of the patient will cause the crosswire image to move, and consequently any attempt at direct measurement of the image size h_1'' will prove difficult and imprecise. The approach to image size measurement in keratometers is to use some type of doubling device and adjust the doubling until the base of one image coincides with the apex of the other. In these circumstances the doubling is equal to the image size.

In *Figure 3.3* the doubling prism is moved along the axis of the telescope (from left to right in the diagram) until the base of the lower image just touches the apex of the upper image. If the prism

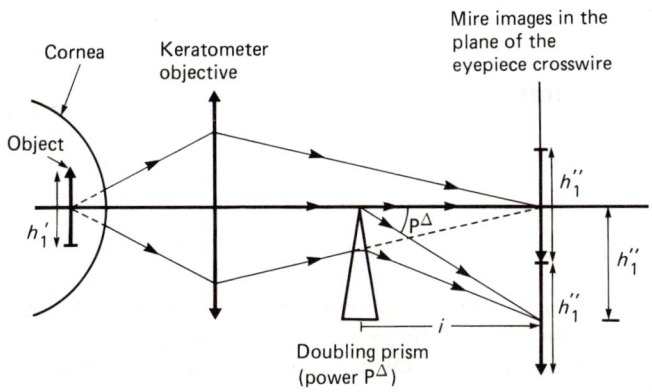

Figure 3.3. The doubling prism.

displacing △ to right, moves image up.

were moved further to the right the images would overlap. With the prism positioned as shown in *Figure 3.3* the doubling of the images (centre to centre) is equal to the image size h_1''.

Prism power $P\Delta$ is defined as the tangent of the angle of deviation multiplied by 100. Thus in *Figure 3.3*

$$P\Delta = \frac{h_1''}{i} \times 100$$

$$\therefore h_1'' = \frac{Pi}{100}$$

Therefore if we know the prism power and the position of the prism we can deduce the size of the image h_1''.

Also from this last equation we can conclude that

$$h_1'' \propto i$$

If we go back to consider the relationship

$$h_1' = \frac{l}{l'} h_1''$$

we can conclude that

$$h_1'' \propto h_1'$$

Therefore

$$h_1' \propto i$$

Finally considering the keratometer equation

$$r = -2\frac{h_1'}{h_1} d$$

we can conclude that

$$r \propto h_1'$$

Therefore

$$r \propto i$$

That is, the movement of the doubling prism is directly proportional to the radius of curvature of the cornea. Therefore the radius scale derived from the doubling prism movement will be a linear scale. This system is called a variable-position doubler.

An alternative option would be to fix the position of the prism and vary its power, giving a variable-power doubler. Since

$$h_1'' = \frac{Pi}{100}$$

once again

$$r \propto P$$

and therefore the radius scale of the keratometer will be linear.

There is, however, another option which involves a fixed amount of doubling in the keratometer telescope with the mire size being altered until the crosswire image size is made equal to the doubling. This is described as a variable-mire-size or fixed-doubling instrument, and the keratometer equation

$$r = -2\frac{h_1'}{h_1}d$$

leads to the conclusion that

$$r \propto \frac{1}{h_1}$$

Therefore the radius scale will not be linear, with crowding occurring for longer radii. However, since the power F is proportional to $1/r$, the corneal power scale will be linear in this type of instrument. Repeat measurement studies on various keratometers suggest that the range of radius values will vary on repeat measurement by around ± 0.05 mm.

3.4 Mire image formation

In *Figure 3.4* the mire is represented as two plus signs which mark the upper and lower extremities of the mire, i.e. the separation of the plus signs gives us the mire size h_1. In making an actual keratometer measurement we superimpose the two extremities and it is therefore only the mire extremities that we are concerned with. The light rays drawn in the diagram illustrate the limiting rays entering the telescope and from these we can see that the corneal image is produced by reflection from only a small eccentric region of the cornea above the axis of the system.

Obviously the lower extremity of the mire will use an identical corneal region below the axis of the system. Thus we can conclude *the two signs represent the extremities; then these can be taken as being the object.*

72 Measurement of the cornea

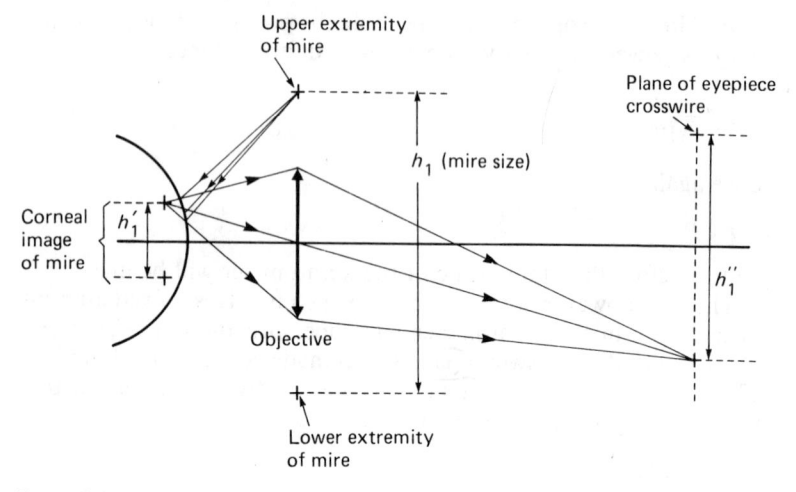

Figure 3.4. The limiting light rays entering the telescope reveal the corneal region involved in producing the mire image.

that the corneal area involved in generating the corneal mire image is an annular region. The size of the annulus will vary according to the instrument characteristics; however, as a generalization we can say that the internal diameter of the annulus is around 2.5 mm with an annulus width of 0.7 mm. This obviously means that the central 2.5 mm of cornea is not involved in producing the mire image. The inner diameter of the annulus can be reduced by reducing the separation of the mire extremities; however, reference to the keratometer equation indicates that this will lower the accuracy of the instrument.

3.5 The telecentric keratometer

Figure 3.5 illustrates the features unique to the telecentric design. The first thing to note is that the mires are collimated so that the corneal image is formed at (rather than near) the focal plane of the cornea. This eliminates the approximation in the keratometer equation (see Section 3.2) since, with the image at the focal point, x equals d due to the collimated system which places the mire at optical infinity. It therefore follows that, as the distance from the mire to the cornea is reduced, the discrepancy between x and d increases owing to the mire image h_1' being displaced from the focal plane of the cornea and this leads to an increase of error in the

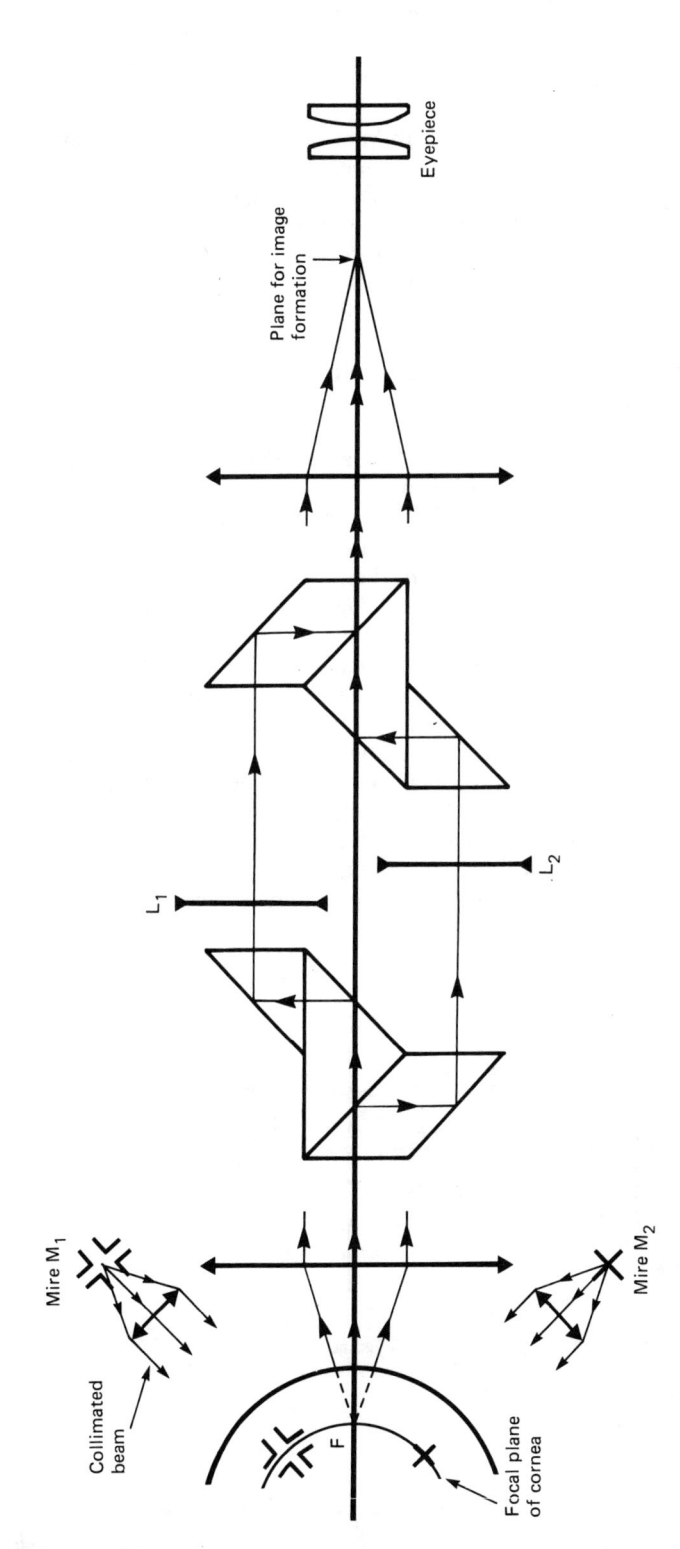

Figure 3.5. The telecentric keratometer. The collimated mire produces an image in the focal plane of the cornea (F). The images from M_1 and M_2 both pass through the two optical systems of the instrument to form two images near the eyepiece. L_1 and L_2 are the prismatic doubling lenses.

equation. In the Bausch and Lomb keratometer where $d = 72$ mm, the error in r is about 0.02 mm. If d is increased to 150 mm the error in r is reduced to around 0.003 mm. Since d is smaller than x then r will acquire a value which is smaller than it should be. Therefore the error above must be added to the keratometer reading acquired.

In *Figure 3.5* the lenses L_1 and L_2 will induce a variable prism power by decentration and so this system uses a variable-power doubler based on this principle. In order to illustrate a major further advantage of the telecentric keratometer it will be necessary to simplify *Figure 3.5*. We will consider what happens to the light passing through the doubling lens L_1.

Figure 3.6 illustrates what happens in a conventional keratometer. When the keratometer is positioned correctly the corneal mire image A will produce an image A' in the plane of the eyepiece crosswire. If the keratometer is positioned too far from the corneal mire image as is the case with the image extremity B, then the image B' formed in the telescope is nearer the objective and *Figure 3.6* illustrates that the image size is reduced. We have established that the keratometer measures the size of this image to deduce the radius of curvature. It is therefore obvious that in a conventional keratometer the examiner must be sure that the eyepiece image is in the plane of the eyepiece crosswire. The best method of doing this is to check that no parallactic displacement of the image relative to the crosswire occurs if the examiner's eye is moved from side to side. If the image and crosswires do not coincide then the radius reading acquired using a standard keratometer will be inaccurate.

The telecentric system is illustrated in *Figure 3.7* where it can be

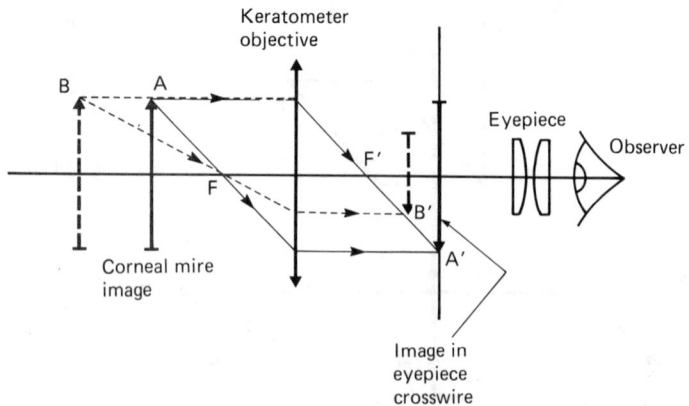

Figure 3.6. Eyepiece image formation.

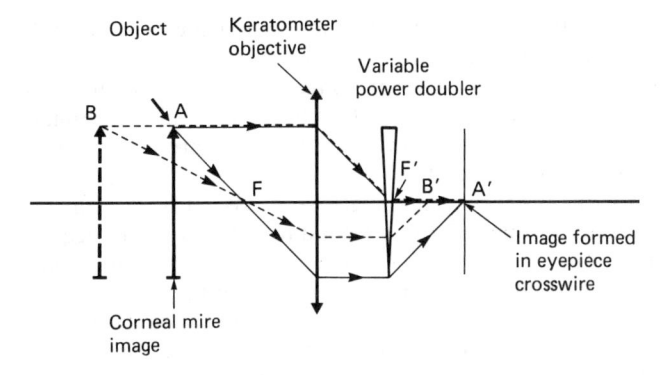

Figure 3.7. The telecentric keratometer.

seen that the variable prism is placed at F' (the principal focus of the keratometer telescope objective). *Figure 3.7* illustrates that, if the keratometer is positioned at an inappropriate distance from the corneal mire image B, the image B' in the telescope—although it may be out of focus due to its being too near the objective—will still lie on the optical axis of the instrument. The mire upper extremity M_1 in *Figure 3.5* is positioned on the axis of the instrument by decentring lens L_1 to give a base-up prism. If the lens L_2 is decentred an identical amount to give a base-down prism then the mire lower extremity M_2 will also lie on the optical axis, i.e. they are superimposed. If the keratometer is then withdrawn from the patient's eye the observed images will defocus but the superimposition will be maintained as illustrated in *Figure 3.7*. We now have a keratometer that does not rely on the observed images being positioned exactly in the plane of the eyepiece crosswire. The telecentric keratometer therefore does not require an adjustable eyepiece or an eyepiece crosswire and is undoubtedly the easiest keratometer to use.

3.6 One- and two-position instruments

A final option open to the designer of a keratometer is the choice between a one- or two-position instrument. In the two-position instrument a single doubling device is used and the keratometer orientation is successively set on each of the two principal meridians of the cornea in order to acquire the anterior corneal radii of these two meridians. In the one-position instrument a pair of doubling devices set mutually at right angles allows a simultaneous measurement of the two principal meridians. However, this is subject to some qualification. The assumption is made that the two principal meridians of the cornea are mutually at right angles and this is not always the case, particularly after prolonged contact lens wear. Also, in the case of a toric cornea the position of the corneal mire images will differ for the two principal meridians. Therefore if one keratometer image is in the plane of the eyepiece crosswire then the image determined by the other principal meridian is not. It is necessary to reposition the keratometer for this second image in order to acquire an accurate value for the radius. In *Figure 3.6* the corneal mire images A and B could be considered to be due to the steep and flat meridians respectively (in fact image B should be a little larger than image A in these circumstances). The radius value acquired from A will be correct because image A' is formed in the eyepiece crosswire. However, the flatter meridian produces an image at B which results in a keratometer image at B' which, as illustrated in *Figure 3.6*, is smaller than it should be. A small image is associated with a short radius of curvature; therefore we can deduce that the corneal radius value acquired will be shorter than if the keratometer were repositioned correctly for this meridian.

For all keratometers the principal meridians are determined by setting the mire images 'in step'. The observation that these images are in step only when the mires are parallel to either of the principal meridians of the cornea arises from the behaviour of light when passing through a toric system. If we consider the 'scissors movement' observed in a toric spectacle lens which is rotated in front of a cross chart then we can relate this to the keratometer, since a mire image moving out of step does so for the same reasons that the two limbs of the cross in a cross chart fail to intersect at 90° when the principal meridians of a toric lens are not horizontal and vertical.

3.7 Extending the range of measurement

There are occasions when the keratometer may be required to measure radii outside the standard range of values, e.g. checking the scleral radii of a scleral contact lens. The range can be extended by using a negative auxiliary lens fixed to the keratometer objective.

In *Figure 3.8(a)* we see a standard keratometer arrangement with the keratometer image h_1'' formed in the plane of the eyepiece crosswire. In *Figure 3.8(b)* the incorporation of a negative auxiliary lens results in a need for the keratometer to be moved further away from the corneal surface in order to ensure that the keratometer image h_2'' is still focussed in the plane of the eyepiece crosswire. The increase in the distance between the mire and the cornea will move

Extending the range of measurement 77

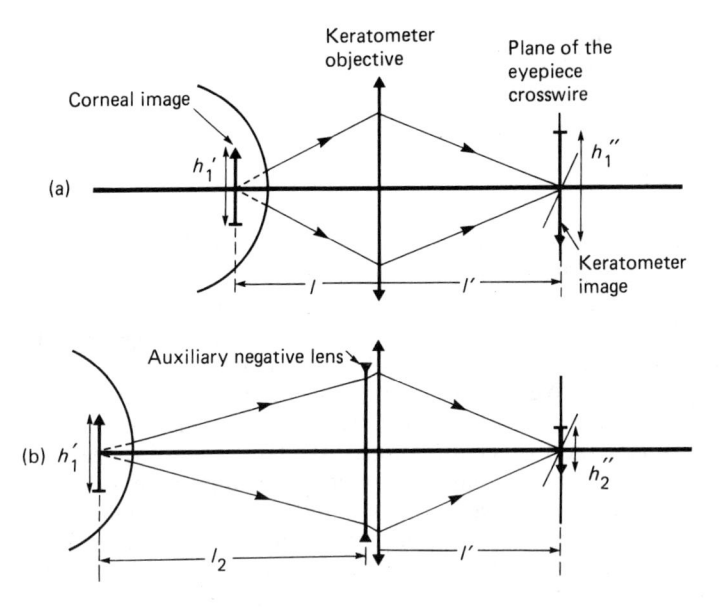

Figure 3.8. (a) The standard keratometer.

Figure 3.8. (b) The same keratometer with a negative auxiliary lens fixed to the keratometer objective.

the corneal image towards the focal plane of the cornea, where it is already assumed to be since we have stated that d equals x in the keratometer equation. What we are really assuming is that the mires represent a distant target and in a telecentric keratometer the mires are at infinity with or without the auxiliary lens. We can conclude that the corneal image h_1' remains unaltered.

If we now consider the relationship

$$\frac{\text{image size}}{\text{object size}} = \frac{\text{image distance}}{\text{object distance}}$$

and substitute in *Figure 3.8(a)* we get

$$\frac{h_1''}{h_1'} = \frac{l'}{l}$$

$$\therefore h_1'' = \frac{l'}{l} h_1'$$

In *Figure 3.8(b)*

$$\frac{h_2''}{h_1'} = \frac{l'}{l_2}$$

$$\therefore h_2'' = \frac{l'}{l_2} h_1'$$

and since l_2 is greater than l then h_2'' must be smaller than h_1''. Thus the negative auxiliary lens has reduced the size of the image in the eyepiece crosswire. A reduction in size of this keratometer image is normally due to a reduction in the size of the corneal image and this is due to a reduction in the radius of curvature of the convex surface being examined. We can therefore conclude that the keratometer with the negative auxiliary lens will read steep. This makes it suitable for measuring radii which are longer than the standard range.

In practice the most convenient method of range extension is to fix the auxiliary lens (power around -1.00 or -2.00 D) in place and measure the radius of ball bearings with the modified keratometer, and then measure the diameter of the ball bearings with a micrometer. This will allow the practitioner to construct a conversion scale.

3.8 The power scale

The keratometer equation allows us to convert the image size into a value for the radius of curvature of the anterior corneal surface. This can be easily converted into dioptric power using the equation

$$F = \frac{n-1}{r}$$

and since the refractive index of the cornea is 1.376 it would seem appropriate to use this as the value for n. However, this indicates the power of the anterior corneal surface only. The total corneal power must include the influence of the posterior corneal surface. If we take the constants of the exact schematic eye as a basis for illustration, then the anterior surface radius is 7.7 mm. With a posterior surface radius of 6.8 mm and a corneal thickness of 0.5 mm, the total vergence change can be calculated by the step along method:

Power of the anterior cornea $F_a = \dfrac{n_c - 1}{r_a} = \dfrac{376}{7.7} = +48.83$ D

Power of the posterior cornea $F_p = \dfrac{n_a - n_c}{r_p} = \dfrac{-40}{6.8} = -5.88$ D

The power scale 79

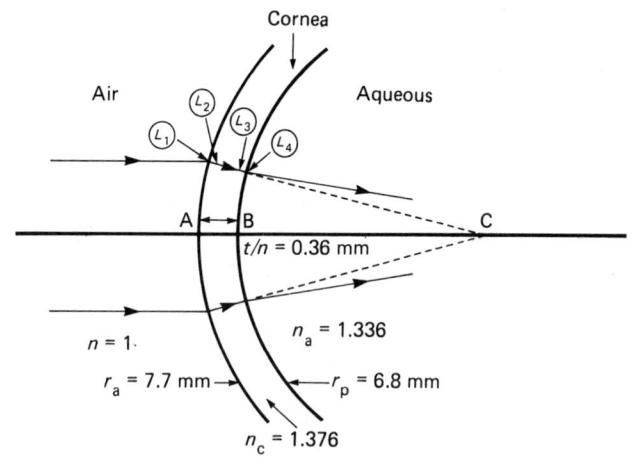

Figure 3.9. The change of vergence of light rays passing through the cornea.

$$\frac{t}{n_c} = \frac{0.5}{1.376} = 0.36 \text{ mm}$$

In *Figure 3.9*

Vergence (D)		Distance (mm)
$L_1 =$ 0.00		
$F_a = +\underline{48.83}$		
$L_2 = +48.83$	$\xrightarrow{\dfrac{1000}{48.83}}$	$20.48 = AC$
		$-\underline{0.36} = t/n$
$L_3 = +49.70$	$\xleftarrow{\dfrac{1000}{20.12}}$	$20.12 = BC$
$F_p = -\underline{5.88}$		
$L_4 = +43.82$		

We can conclude that the total vergence change for light from a point source at infinity passing through this cornea is $+43.82$ D which is the BVP of the cornea.

If we now go back to use the equation $F = (n-1)/r$ but substitute in that equation the total power of the cornea with the radius of the anterior cornea, we obtain a refractive index which can be used to predict total corneal power having measured the radius of curvature of only the anterior corneal surface:

$n - 1 = Fr = 43.82 \times 0.0077$

$n = 1.3375$

Therefore, if we use a refractive index of 1.3375 to convert anterior corneal surface radius into dioptric power, then the power acquired will be that of the total cornea (anterior and posterior surfaces), provided the cornea under examination has similar characteristics to the exact schematic eye. The dioptric power reported by the keratometer must thus be viewed with caution. If there is a 2.00 D difference between the principal meridians of a toric cornea according to the keratometer, we can only conclude that the approximate total corneal astigmatism is 2.00 D. In the past, some instrument manufacturers have used refractive index values other than 1.3375 and so different instruments may indicate slightly different corneal power values for the same corneal radius. Zeiss, for example, assume the refractive index to be 1.332. American Optical use 1.336 as the refractive index value.

If the keratometer power scale has been constructed using $n = 1.3375$ then a radius of 7.5 mm gives a power reading of 45 D.

One final point to note from the constants of the exact schematic eye is that the ratio of corneal posterior to anterior surface power is $5.88/48.83 = 0.12$. This means that the posterior surface power is approximately 12% of the anterior surface power. The ratio is often rounded down to 1/10 for convenience.

3.9 The keratometer used to check concave surfaces

The equations encountered in this chapter are derived assuming paraxial theory. Emsley (1963) and Bennett (1966) have shown this to be an over-simplification. The corneal areas from which the mire images are reflected are too far from the axis of the system to be considered as being in the paraxial region of a surface of reflecting power -260 D. Bennett (1966) has shown that the difference in the aberrations of convex and concave surfaces can account for the corrections which have to be applied when a keratometer is used to measure the BCOR of a contact lens, whereas the paraxial formulae apply equally to concave and convex surfaces. The error is about 0.02 mm for steep radii (6.50 mm) and around 0.04 mm for flat radii

(9.50 mm). For most of the BCORs encountered in contact lens work it is sufficient to add 0.03 mm to the radius given by the instrument.

3.10 Precautions

The keratometer is an image size measuring device. It is therefore essential (with the exception of the telecentric keratometer) to have this image in the plane of the eyepiece crosswire. When using a keratometer:

(1) Turn the eyepiece anticlockwise. Look through the telescope at a distant object and turn the eyepiece clockwise until the crosswire first comes into focus. The crosswire is now at your far point.
(2) Start the measurement with the instrument distant to the cornea and approach the cornea with the instrument until the mire images first come into focus. The mire images are now at your far point.
(3) During the time that the mire images are being made to coincide, the practitioner should see the crosswire and mire images clearly simultaneously. If they are not simultaneously clear the mire images are not in the same plane as the eyepiece crosswire. The instrument position must be constantly adjusted to maintain the necessary picture. Therefore, when superimposing the mire images, one hand must be on the joystick adjusting the instrument position while the other hand is used to superimpose the mire images.
(4) The power scale uses an assumed refractive index which allows prediction of the total corneal astigmatism from a measurement of anterior surface radius of curvature. The power scale must therefore be used with this in mind.
(5) The keratometer error arising from the mires being near the cornea increases if the instrument is designed to operate near the eye, i.e. where d or x in the keratometer equation has a small value.
(6) The mire images are formed by an annular area of some 3 mm diameter. The keratometer therefore is indicating radius of curvature of this area and this area only.

3.11 The topographic keratometer

If we return to Section 3.4 we can see in *Figure 3.4* that, when taking a keratometric measurement of the central cornea, the image is produced by two corneal regions approximately 0.7 mm in diameter and 1.6 mm from the corneal vertex. If the visual axis of the eye in *Figure 3.4* is directed inferiorly then the light rays from the lower extremity of the mire may well strike the cornea at or near its apex. At the same time the light rays from the upper extremity of the mire would be reflected by a section of the anterior cornea near the upper limbus. The lower mire extremity image will be formed by the central cornea with the upper extremity formed by the flatter periphery. Any reading taken in these circumstances is of questionable value.

Essentially the problem described above arises from the mire size h_1 being too large. We could measure the radius of curvature of the peripheral corneal regions if we reduced the size of the mire, and this is the approach adopted in the topographic keratometer. If in the circumstances described we switch off the lower mire extremity and regard the upper extremity as the entire mire, then the corneal image is formed by the peripheral corneal region only. We then simply need to double the extremity to measure its size. This inevitably requires a considerably weaker doubling device.

The disadvantage of a small mire can be seen when the keratometer equation is examined. A small value for h_1 means that a smaller change in image size h_1' will occur for any given change in radius. Thus the precision of keratometric measurement is reduced due to reduced sensitivity of the instrument arising from a small mire size. Therefore the central keratometer reading is taken by 'classical keratometry', with the small mire size being used for peripheral radius measurement only. The eccentric measurements are made by displacing the fixation spot from the optical axis of the instrument. It must be noted that the eye rotates about the centre of rotation of the sclera and this results in the cornea being tilted with increasing eccentricity. Thus the examiner must laterally shift the position of the keratometer when making peripheral radius measurements along the horizontal meridian.

The topographic keratometer should not be confused with the topogometer which is simply a movable fixation device attached to a standard keratometer. The fixation device is displaced from the optical axis of the instrument until the observed image starts to change size. It is thus simply a means of assessing the diameter of the corneal cap, i.e. the central area of the cornea over which there is no appreciable change in radius of curvature.

3.12 The photokeratoscope

It will be recalled from Section 3.4 that the corneal region used to generate the mire image is approximately 1.6 mm from the vertex. If in *Figure 3.4* the mire size h_1 is increased, then the corneal region involved is made even more eccentric. This is the underlying principle of the photokeratoscope. The mire is replaced by a set of concentric circles of increasing diameter. The size of the corneal image of the small central circle can be used to calculate the radius of curvature of the central cornea, whereas the corneal image of the largest circle is used to calculate the radius of curvature of the corneal periphery. The image size is measured from a photograph of the anterior eye. Criticisms of this approach are that:

(1) Film shrinkage may occur during development.
(2) The orientation of the principal meridians is not obvious.
(3) The film grain inevitably means that the edges of the image will show some blurring under magnified inspection.

However, photokeratoscopes have been used successfully in practice and possess the significant advantage of assessing the topography of the cornea. A typical modern system consists of seven concentric circles which are used to analyse the cornea in 1 mm increments from a diameter of 3 mm to 9 mm. The image plane for these circles must be flat if all seven circles are to be focussed on the camera film simultaneously. The arrangement of the circles will depend on the topography of the surface under examination and so some sort of assumptions about the surface will have to be made. The circles are usually arranged so that their loci form an ellipsoid as shown in *Figure 3.10*.

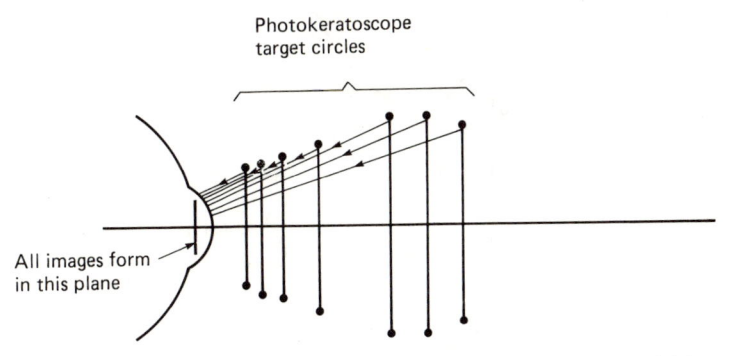

Figure 3.10. The positions and sizes of the seven concentric targets which produce an image by reflection in the cornea in a flat plane.

84 Measurement of the cornea

The ellipsoidal target surface will theoretically produce a flat image plane when the light is reflected from a spherical surface of specified radius, and this is a further criticism of the instrument since the accuracy will deteriorate as the reflecting surface deviates from the standard form. Reproducibility studies claim a maximum standard deviation from the mean of 0.01 mm; however, this applies to measurement of an accurately known spherical steel ball.

A toric cornea will produce elliptical rather than circular images and the principal meridians are revealed by the long axis (flat meridian) and short axis (steep meridian) of the ellipse, but of course the image cannot form in a plane in these circumstances.

3.13 The pachometer

The pachometer is an instrument which, in conjunction with a slit lamp, measures the apparent thickness of the cornea. Its working principles are illustrated in *Figure 3.11*, where the eye under examination fixates the slit beam which therefore passes approximately through the corneal apex. The observer views the optical section by using the biomicroscope set at the specified angle θ. The observed thickness of the cornea in these circumstances is BE. From *Figure 3.11* we can deduce that

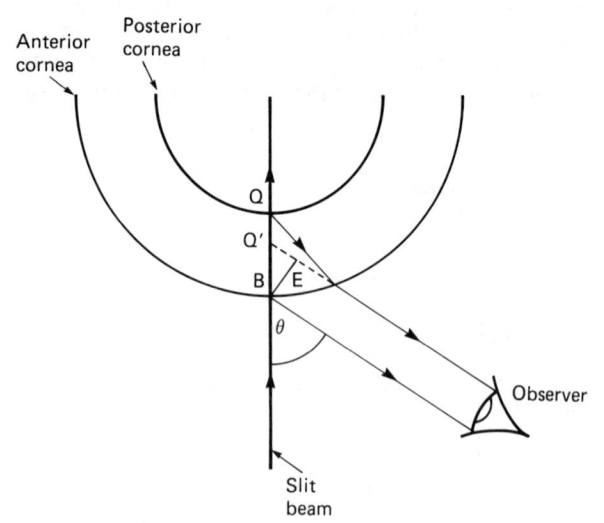

Figure 3.11. The optical section observed during a pachometric measurement. The biomicroscope has been omitted for simplicity.

$$BQ' = \frac{BE}{\sin \theta}$$

and BQ' is the apparent thickness. The instrument scale is calibrated to read apparent thickness, and this can be converted to real thickness by reference to tables supplied with the instrument which take corneal radius of curvature into account. As with keratometry we must devise some means of measuring the size of BE and once again a doubling system is incorporated into the instrument. This consists of a thick glass plate placed into the observation system. Half of the aperture is covered by a fixed plate, the other half by a plate which can be tilted as shown in *Figure 3.12*. This provides an

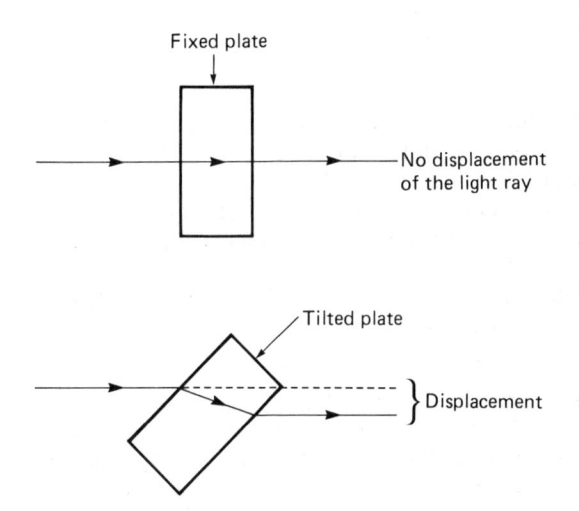

Figure 3.12. Light ray displacement by tilting a thick glass plate.

ability to displace half the image of the optical section as shown in *Figure 3.13*. The fixed plate is included in the system so that the length of the optical path in the two halves of the system does not differ significantly. The end point is reached when the posterior corneal surface of one half of the aperture coincides with the anterior corneal surface of the other.

3.13.1 Precautions

(1) The illuminating beam must be normal to the corneal surface. This is best confirmed by asking the patient to look at the light

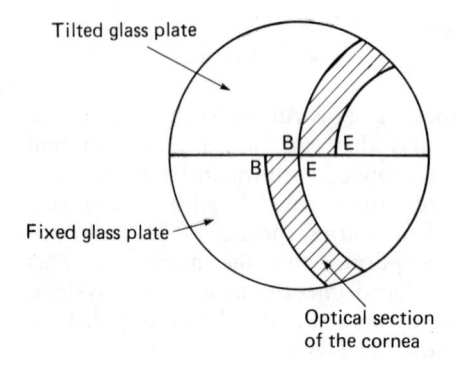

Figure 3.13. The optical section appearance when the pachometer is set to measure apparent corneal thickness.

source and checking that the reflected light returns to the slit aperture of the pachometer. This requires a small screen mounted just above the slit aperture.
(2) Vertical alignment is best achieved by bisecting the first Purkinje image with the dividing line between the upper and lower glass plates.
(3) As with any optical section the slit beam should be as narrow as possible, with the light source as bright as possible to help compensate for the light loss.

With some instruments the observation is always made to the right of the slit beam. This means an observation on the nasal side of the apex for a right eye and the temporal side for a left. This has been suggested as the cause for the significant differences observed between right and left eyes in a number of investigations.

4 The cornea and contact lens combination

4.1 Corneal topography

The corneal topography is not easily assessed and in consequence has been a topic of contention in the past. The more recent investigations appear to suggest that the cornea is elliptical in form with a *p* value around 0.8 in an average eye. It may come as a surprise that Helmholtz in his book *Physiological Optics* described the cornea as an ellipsoid. Helmholtz examined the corneas of three subjects and his results can be used to calculate *p* which comes out as 0.56, 0.76 and 0.7 for these three individuals.

Recent investigations have revealed that the *p* value can vary considerably in the normal population. Unfortunately at the moment there is no convenient clinical method for determining the corneal topography and so any consideration of the relationship between a contact lens and the cornea on which it rests must start with some assumptions about the cornea. In fact, the Wesley–Jessen system 2000 photokeratoscope provides enough information to calculate the *p* value of the cornea, but it is the only clinical instrument that performs this function at the moment.

4.2 Tear lens thickness and edge clearance

One possible approach to achieving an optimum relationship between the contact lens and the cornea, suggested by Townsley (1970), is to ensure an optimum value for the axial tear lens thickness (TLT) at the cornea/contact lens vertex.

According to Guillon *et al.* (1983) this should be around 0.02 mm. Tomlinson and Bibby (1977) concluded that the optimum value is 0.015 mm. The edge clearance from the cornea is also considered in a similar way. Tomlinson and Bibby (1977) recommend a radial edge clearance of 0.08 mm (measured normal to the cornea). Guillon *et al.* (1983) proposed 0.08 mm axial edge clearance (which approximates to 0.07 mm radial clearance). Atkinson (1984) considers

0.08 mm axial edge clearance to be optimum for gas permeable lenses, with the 0.08 mm radial edge clearance being somewhat excessive.

Any fitting set designed to incorporate the concept of constant TLT or edge clearance will be based on a particular corneal form. This inevitably means that in individual patients with atypical corneas the TLT or edge clearance will not meet the expected value.

4.3 Calculation of TLT and edge clearance

The relationship between the contact lens and the cornea is illustrated in *Figure 4.1*. The sags in this diagram can be calculated by using the equations derived in Sections 2.10–2.13. *Figure 4.1* illustrates that we need only concern ourselves with the sag of the contact lens and that of the anterior cornea. The TLT can be deduced from the relationship

$$AB = AC - BC$$

where AB equals the TLT, AC is the sag of the contact lens over semi-diameter y_1, and BC is the sag of the cornea over semi-diameter y_1.

The edge clearance can be calculated from

$$DE = AB + BE - AD$$

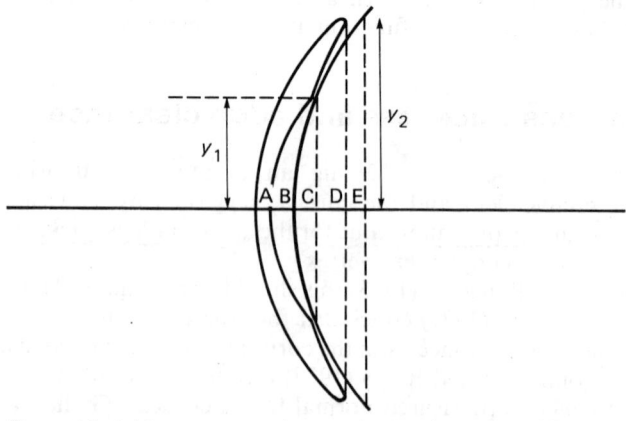

Figure 4.1. A bicurve contact lens resting on the cornea. AB is the central tear layer thickness TLT. DE is the axial edge clearance. AD is the primary sag of the contact lens. BE is the primary sag of the cornea.

where DE is the edge clearance, AB is the TLT, BE is the primary sag of the anterior cornea over semi-diameter y_2, and AD is the primary sag of the contact lens over semi-diameter y_2.

Although *Figure 4.1* illustrates a bicurve contact lens, the above treatment can be applied to multicurve, offset bicurve or aspheric lenses provided that the primary sag over semi-diameter y_2 and the point of contact between the lens and the cornea (which defines y_1) are known. This latter point is often taken as the BCOD which solves the problem for all but the aspheric lenses. A computer program is presented in Chapter 7 which calculates TLT and axial edge clearance from the cornea after the lens specification has been entered.

4.4 Corneal astigmatism

Taking the constants of the exact schematic eye as a basis for illustration and supposing that the anterior corneal radius is correct in the horizontal meridian (7.7 mm) but 10% shorter in the vertical meridian (6.93 mm), then the dioptric power of the anterior corneal surface will be +48.83 D along 180 and +54.26 D along 90; this gives 5.43 D of anterior surface astigmatism, with the rule, i.e. the vertical meridian is more positive than the horizontal by 5.43 D. However, if the back surface of the cornea is also assumed to be toroidal in form with the same principal meridians, the horizontal meridian radius will be 6.8 mm (exact eye) with the vertical meridian radius 10% shorter, giving a radius value of 6.12 mm. The dioptric power of the posterior corneal surface is deduced using the relationship

$$\text{power} = \frac{n_a - n_c}{r}$$

where n_a and n_c are the refractive indices of the aqueous and cornea respectively. The dioptric power of the horizontal meridian is −5.88 D and the vertical meridian is −6.54 D, giving 0.66 D of against-the-rule astigmatism, i.e. the vertical meridian is more negative than the horizontal by 0.66 D. Therefore the anterior surface astigmatism of 5.43 D is reduced to a total corneal astigmatism of

$$5.43 - 0.66 = 4.77 \text{ D}$$

(assuming the cornea is thin). Thus the total corneal astigmatism is approximately 90% of the anterior corneal astigmatism. When a spherical back surface hard or GPH (gas permeable) contact lens rests on the eye, the toric cornea has some of its anterior surface astigmatism neutralized by the fluid lens. The fluid lens in these circumstances has a spherical front surface and a toric back surface and so it is obviously the back surface of the fluid lens which is responsible for the astigmatic neutralization. The amount of dioptric power, and therefore the amount of astigmatism neutralized, can be deduced from the relationship

$$F_C \text{ for the anterior cornea} = \frac{1.376-1}{r_c}$$

$$F_F \text{ for the posterior surface of the fluid lens} = \frac{1.336-1}{r_c}$$

where r_c is the corneal radius. The ratio of fluid surface power to corneal surface power F_F/F_C is therefore 336/376, i.e. the ratio of the refractivities which approximates to 9/10. Thus approximately nine-tenths of the anterior corneal surface astigmatism is neutralized by the back surface of the fluid lens. It will be recalled that the posterior surface of the cornea neutralizes the remaining one-tenth approximately. We can therefore conclude that a spherical back surface contact lens fitted to a toric cornea will, by means of the accompanying fluid lens, neutralize the corneal astigmatism. Once again note that this is independent of the refractive index of the contact lens.

4.5 Residual astigmatism

When an eye is fitted with spherical back surface hard or GPH contact lens, the corneal astigmatism is neutralized and the wearer can attain a high level of visual acuity with only a spherical power. However, in some cases the contact lens over-refraction reveals the presence of astigmatism. This astigmatism must arise from eye components other than the cornea and is therefore most probably due to the crystalline lens. This astigmatism still present during the contact lens over-refraction using spherical lenses is called residual astigmatism and from the foregoing could also be called lenticular astigmatism. These terms can often therefore be used synonymously. Thus

residual astigmatism = total ocular astigmatism minus the corneal astigmatism

or

residual astigmatism = total ocular astigmatism minus the astigmatism measured by the keratometer

An astigmatic effect is created when the chief ray of an incident pencil does not coincide with the optical axis, and so a decentred contact lens may well produce apparent residual astigmatism. It is therefore important to ensure a well centred lens at the time of the over-refraction.

A soft lens (particularly a thin soft lens) will align itself to the anterior cornea and this means that its surfaces will take up the same toricity as the cornea on which the contact lens is resting. This results in the lens transmitting all the corneal astigmatism and thus in these circumstances the residual astigmatism is approximately equal to the ocular astigmatism. Soft lens manufacturers claim that, with thicker and lower water content soft lenses, some of the corneal astigmatism is neutralized; however, the total ocular astigmatism needs to be less than 1.00 D unless the wearer is prepared to accept some significant visual blur with a spherical soft lens.

The practitioner may occasionally encounter a patient with a spherical refractive error but with a toric cornea. The theoretical implication here is that the corneal astigmatism is neutralized by the lenticular astigmatism. If this patient is fitted with a spherical back surface hard or GPH lens, then the corneal astigmatism is neutralized, leaving the residual lenticular astigmatism manifest. A spherical correction worked onto this contact lens would result in a visual acuity poorer than that obtained with spectacles. A soft lens, on the other hand, will transmit most of the corneal astigmatism which will therefore maintain neutralization of the lenticular astigmatism, resulting in a good visual acuity.

4.6 Back surface toric lenses

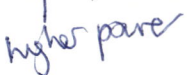

Increasing corneal toricity ultimately leads to a situation where a spherical back surface contact lens will not be tolerated by the wearer. In these circumstances the fitting relationship between the cornea and the contact lens may be improved by using a toric back surface contact lens. The general approach for hard and GPH lenses appears to be to use a lens which aligns with the flatter corneal meridian and fits slightly flat on the steeper meridian. The fluorescein picture will be similar to that observed when a spherical back surface lens is resting on a slightly toric cornea. The disadvantage of a toric back surface contact lens is that the fluid lens will no longer correct the corneal astigmatism since it now has a toric front surface. Essentially, on the steeper meridian, the anterior surface of the fluid lens becomes more positive and the back surface of the contact lens becomes more negative when a change is made from a spherical to a toric contact lens. The contact lens refractive index is higher than that of the tears and this therefore results in over-correction of the corneal astigmatism, since the fluid lens anterior surface becomes more positive but the contact lens back surface becomes more negative, and this change is the greater as the BCOR is reduced on the steeper corneal meridian. We can therefore conclude that the fitting of a toric back surface contact lens will result in induced astigmatism manifesting itself. This induced astigmatism is present at the contact lens/fluid lens interface. The induced astigmatism can be neutralized by producing a toric front surface, and the contact lens then becomes a parallel bitoric lens. In these circumstances the toric front surface is there to correct the induced astigmatism and so, when the contact lens rotates on the eye, the induced astigmatism and its correcting surface maintain their alignment which results in no visual deterioration in clarity.

It may be useful at this stage to take a typical example:

ocular refraction   −1.00 DS/−3.00 DC × 180

keratometry readings   8.10 along 180; 7.55 along 90

The keratometry readings suggest that the astigmatism is corneal. A contact lens fitting session indicates that a toric lens is required for ocular comfort; however, only a spherical fitting set is available. The lens which provides an alignment fit along 180 is

    C2   8.10:6.50/8.70:9.00   BVP −0.50 DS

The over-refraction result with this lens is −0.50 DS, giving a visual acuity of 6/5. The lack of any cylinder and the high visual acuity support the notion that this astigmatism is corneal.

The practitioner decides to order a toric back surface with BCORs of 8.10 mm along 180 and 7.7 mm along 90. The BVP for this specification is calculated as follows.

Along 180

The fitting relationship is illustrated in *Figure 4.2*. The over-refraction result indicates that the contact lens BVP must be −1.00 DS to correct the refractive error of this meridian. The specification for this meridian remains unchanged in the lens to be ordered since the BCOR is still 8.10 mm. Therefore the BVP to be ordered remains unaltered at −1.00 DS.

Along 90

In *Figure 4.3* the over-refraction with the fitting set lens indicated a

Back surface toric lenses 93

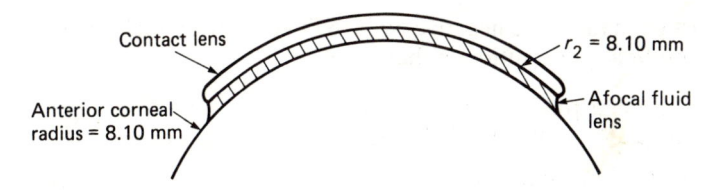

Figure 4.2. The fitting relationship along the 180 meridian.

BVP required of $-0.50 - 0.50 = -1.00$ DS. However, in the toric lens to be ordered (*Figure 4.3(b)*) the BCOR is reduced from 8.10 mm to 7.7 mm. The diagrams illustrate that this makes the fluid lens less negative in power. A BCOR of 7.7 mm gives an anterior surface power to the fluid lens in air of

$$\frac{336}{7.7} = +43.64 \text{ D}$$

A BCOR of 8.1 mm gives an anterior surface power to the fluid lens in air of

$$\frac{336}{8.1} = +41.48 \text{ D}$$

∴ Fluid lens anterior surface astigmatism = 2.16 D

We can conclude that along the 90 meridian the fluid lens is 2.16 D more positive than at the time of the over-refraction.

If the contact lens is to maintain a correction identical with that of the spherical lens used for the over-refraction, then its power along

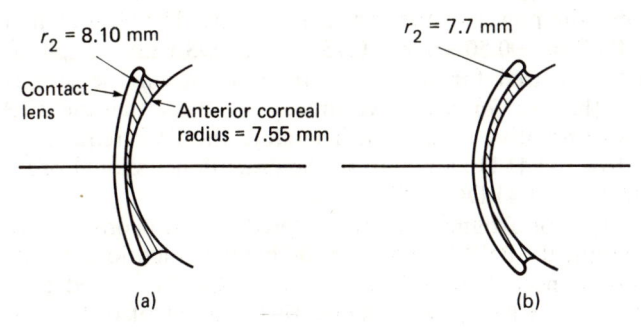

Figure 4.3. The fitting relationship along the 90 meridian, (a) using the spherical fitting set lens, and (b) using the toric lens.

90 must be made more negative by 2.16 D at the back surface of the lens. The final prescription is therefore:

C2 $\genfrac{}{}{0pt}{}{\text{parallel}}{\text{bitoric}} \dfrac{8.10}{7.7}$ m 180 : 6.50 $\dfrac{8.70}{8.30}$: 9.00
− 1.00 DS/ − 2.16 DC × 180

[handwritten note: must be 0.4 mm difference]

It is likely that the 2.16 D would be rounded to the nearest 0.25 D.

In fact, the reduction in BCOR from 8.1 mm to 7.7 mm will induce a back surface cylinder on the contact lens which is 3.14 D, again confirming over-correction of the astigmatism; so the contact lens will have a front surface where the vertical meridian is steeper than the horizontal in order to achieve the BVP requested.

If yet again we go back to the approximate rule on change of fluid lens power, i.e. 0.1 mm radius change induces 0.50 D power change, we can consider its application to the above example. We know that the horizontal meridian requires a BVP of − 1.00 D. The lens radius is to be reduced by 0.4 mm in the vertical meridian. The approximate rule tells us that this will induce a power change in the fluid lens of + 2.00 D. The contact lens power must be made more negative by 2.00 D to compensate. Therefore the BVP requested would be − 1.00 DS/ − 2.00 DC × 180. Once again the approximate rule serves us very well and the use of simple mental arithmetic means that it is ideal for clinical work. The accuracy can be improved by using a Heine's table or scale.

If in the above example there had been some residual astigmatism which became apparent at the over-refraction, then the approach to the problem remains unaltered. For example, suppose the over-refraction result in the above example had been − 0.50 DS/ + 0.75 DC × 180. The 180 meridian as before still requires a BVP of − 0.50 − 0.50 = − 1.00 DS, i.e. the power of the sphere in the refractor head plus the power of the trial contact lens. The 90 meridian requires a BVP of − 0.50 − 0.50 + 0.75 = − 0.25 DS with the spherical contact lens used for the over-refraction. When the lens is converted to the toric form we have already calculated that the BVP must be more negative by 2.16 D. Therefore the BVP required is − 0.25 − 2.16 = − 2.41 D along 90, so the practitioner should order BVP − 1.00 DS/ − 1.41 DC × 180.

Thus the type of astigmatism encountered is of no consequence when calculating the BVP. The only thing that the practitioner needs to retain is the concept that, if the contact lens BCOR is altered, then this induces a fluid lens power change of the order of 0.50 D for every 0.1 mm change in radius. Where residual astigmatism is present, either alone or in combination with corneal astigmatism, then the contact lens must maintain its orientation if it is to correct fully the refractive error.

4.7 Front surface toric lenses

If we consider an eye with a spherical cornea which is fitted with a spherical back surface contact lens and is then subjected to an over-refraction, we may find that the best visual acuity is only achieved when a cylindrical element is added to the over-refraction. We have discovered the presence of residual or lenticular astigmatism which will need correcting.

If the back surface of the contact lens is made toric then this will serve to make the lens less comfortable, and it is difficult to imagine any reason for fitting a spherical cornea with a toric back surface lens. The most obvious way of overcoming the problem is to order a toric front surface for the contact lens. Let us take an example:

Ocular refraction	-2.50 DS$/-1.50$ DC $\times$ 90
Keratometry readings	7.80 mm spherical
Trial contact lens C2	7.80:6.50/8.30:9.00 BVP -2.00
Over-refraction	-0.50 DS$/-1.50$ DC $\times$ 90
Visual acuity	6/5

In this case the contact lens BVP to be ordered will be -2.50 DS$/-1.50$ DC $\times$ 90 for a contact lens BCOR of 7.80 mm. A toric front surface will be required, and so it may be more appropriate to consider the positive sphere cyl form -4.00 DS$/+1.50$ DC $\times$ 180. This tells us that the front surface of the contact lens must incorporate a positive cylinder axis 180 and its power will be a little less than 1.50 DC (the contact lens is thick). Let us suppose the central thickness of the lens to be ordered is 0.2 mm. What front surface radii are required for this lens?

We can deal with the two principal meridians as though they were separate lenses.

Along 180
The BVP required for the contact lens for this meridian is $-2.00 - 0.50 - 1.50 = -4.00$ D. Thus in *Figure 4.4* the vergence L_4 must be -4.00 D.

Back surface power $F_2 = \dfrac{-490}{7.8} = -62.82$ D

Reduced thickness $t/n = 0.2/1.490 = 0.13$ mm

96 The cornea and contact lens combination

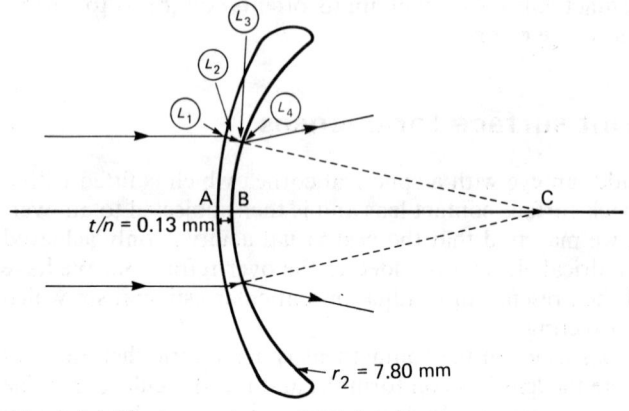

Figure 4.4. The contact lens to be ordered.

      Vergence (D)   *Distance (mm)*

$L_4 = -4.00$

$F_2 = -62.82$

$L_3 = +58.82 \xrightarrow{\dfrac{1000}{+58.82}} 17 = BC$

$\phantom{L_3 = +58.82 \xrightarrow{\dfrac{1000}{+58.82}}\ } 0.13 = t/n$

$L_2 = +58.37 \xleftarrow{\dfrac{1000}{17.13}} 17.13 = AC$

$L_1 = 00.00$

$F_1 = +58.37$

$r_1 = \dfrac{490}{+58.37} = 8.39 \text{ mm} \ \checkmark$

Along 90

The BVP required for the contact lens for this meridian is $-2.00 - 0.50 = -2.50$ D. Thus in *Figure 4.4* the vergence L_4 must be -2.50 D. The back surface power F_2 is, as before, -62.82 D and the reduced thickness is 0.13 mm.

Front surface toric lenses 97

Vergence (D)   *Distance (mm)*

$L_4 = -2.50$

$F_2 = -62.82$

$L_3 = +60.32 \xrightarrow{\quad \frac{1000}{+60.32} \quad} 16.58 = BC$

$\qquad\qquad\qquad\qquad\qquad\qquad 0.13 = t/n$

$L_2 = +59.84 \xleftarrow{\quad \frac{1000}{16.71} \quad} 16.71 = AC$

$L_1 = 0.00$

$F_1 = +59.84$

$r_1 = \dfrac{490}{+59.84} = 8.19 \text{ mm}$

Therefore the front surface radii for this lens are 8.39 mm along 180 and 8.19 mm along 90. This toric front surface is correcting the residual astigmatism and it is therefore imperative that the lens maintain its orientation. We must incorporate an element in the lens which endows it with some rotational stability. The popular solutions to this problem are to use: a heavy metal plug at the lens periphery which acts as ballast; a prism worked on the lens which again has a ballasting effect; or a single or double truncation which in conjunction with the lid margins may produce rotational stability. In the prism-ballasted lens the maximum prism power likely to be tolerated by the eye is 3 Δ and it may be preferable to go for a slightly lower value of 2 Δ. With all three approaches the lens may not behave as expected, i.e. the lens may not adopt an orientation with the metal plug directly below the geometric centre of the lens; or the prism base apex line vertical; or the truncations horizontal. It is therefore advisable to insert appropriate lenses in order to observe the likely orientation adopted by the lens on any particular eye.

4.7.1 Specifying the orientation

In *Figure 4.5* we see a contact lens which has settled to a truncation orientation of 15. The toric front surface of this lens will be calculated from the over-refraction measurements which are given in standard notation. However, the lens manufacturer must relate the principal meridians of the front surface to the truncation line which is expected to take up a horizontal orientation. The lens in *Figure 4.5* has rotated 15° in an anticlockwise direction from this ideal. This serves to increase the orientation value (using standard notation) of both the truncation and the toric surface principal meridians. If we wish to restore the toric surface back to a correct orientation we must reduce the orientation value in relation to the truncation line by 15°. If, for example, we required a lens of BVP -2.00 DS/ $+1.50$ DC $\times 25$ then we would order the $+1.50$ DC at axis 10 to the truncation line, since this itself is already at 15. This reasoning results in an easily remembered rule:

- If the lens rotates anticlockwise, then subtract the degree of rotation from the standard notation orientation of the cylinder.
- If the lens rotates clockwise, then add the degree of rotation to the standard notation orientation of the cylinder.

The only problem that remains is that of accurately assessing the orientation of the truncation on the eye. This is best achieved by placing a well adjusted trial frame on the face with a low powered full aperture cylindrical trial case lens clipped into the cylindrical cell. This type of lens is clearly marked with its axis, and also has two crescent-shaped frosted glass areas at the lens periphery whose straight edges are parallel to the cylinder axis. The cylinder is rotated until these lines are parallel to the truncation and the cylinder axis orientation can be read off the protractor scale on the trial frame.

The above approach applies also to a ballasted lens which will be marked either with the vertical ballast line or a line at right angles to this.

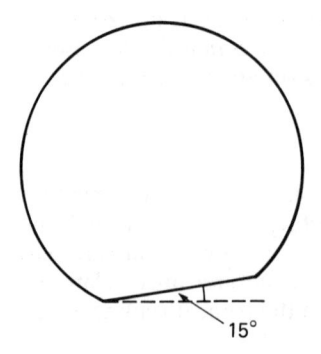

Figure 4.5. A truncated contact lens which has settled with the truncation lying along the 15° meridian.

4.8 The fitting relationship on a toric cornea

If a practitioner is attempting to fit a moderately toric cornea with a spherical back surface hard or GPH contact lens, then a commonly encountered recommendation is to use a BCOR somewhere between the radii of the two principal meridians of the cornea as measured by the keratometer. The usual recommendation is to go for a BCOR one-third of the way from the flatter meridian, two-thirds from the steeper. For example, if the keratometer readings were

   7.90 along 180 : 7.30 along 90

then a contact lens of BCOR 7.7 mm may represent the best compromise fit. This lens is a little steep along 180 and is flat along 90 but not as flat as would be the case if a BCOR of 7.90 mm (aligning with the 180 meridian) is used. It is claimed that the 7.7 mm lens results in a reduced edge standoff at the top and bottom of the lens. Some workers have disputed this, claiming that since the lens is steep along 180 this lifts the lens vertex off the corneal apex, which restores the edge clearance to much the same value as a lens which is fitted on alignment with the 180 meridian. <u>Let us take an example.</u>

A cornea with vertex radii of 7.90 mm along 180 and 7.30 mm along 90 and a p value of 0.8 is fitted with a bicurve lens of the following specification:

   C2   7.90:7.00/10.50:8.50

(1) What is the axial edge clearance along 90?
(2) What would the edge clearance be along 90 if the contact lens BCOR was changed to 7.7 mm with the other lens parameters unchanged?

We must make the usual assumption that the contact lens touches the cornea at the BCOD transition.

(1) C2   7.90:7.00/10.50:8.50

Along 180

The cornea

   $r_0 = 7.90$ mm, $p = 0.8$

   $x_{180} = \dfrac{r_0}{p} - \sqrt{\left(\dfrac{r_0}{p}\right)^2 - \dfrac{y_1^2}{p}}$ (from Section 2.12)

   $x_{180} = 0.808$ mm for diameter 7.00 mm

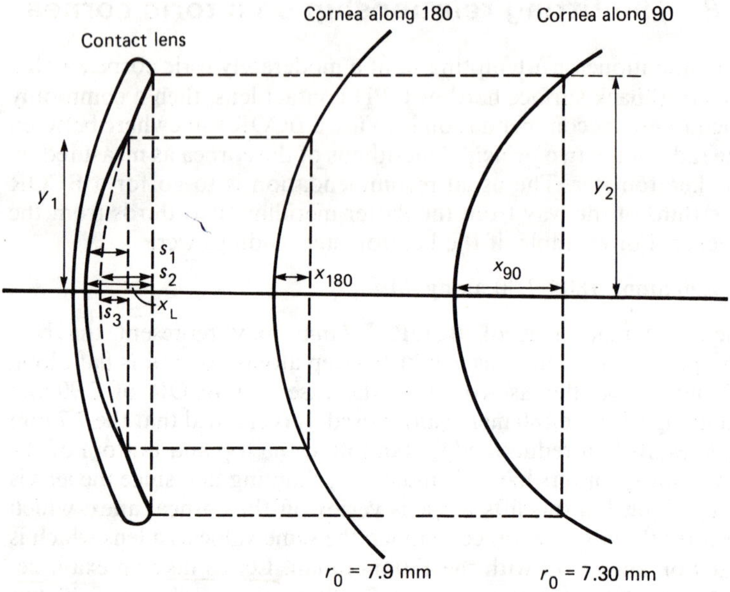

Figure 4.6. The C2 contact lens and the two anterior corneal principal meridians.

The contact lens
The sag s_1 is 0.818 mm for diameter 7.00 mm (using the sag equation in Section 2.10). $s = r - \sqrt{r^2 - y^2}$ where $r = 7.90$, $y = 3.50$.

TLT
In Section 4.3 we deduced that

TLT = sag of contact lens s_1 − primary sag of cornea x_{180}
TLT = 0.818 − 0.808 = 0.01 mm

Along 90

The TLT is 0.01 mm.

The cornea
$r_0 = 7.3$ mm, $p = 0.8$

$$x_{90} = \frac{r_0}{p} - \sqrt{\left(\frac{r_0}{p}\right)^2 - \frac{y_2^2}{p}}$$ from Section 2.12

$x_{90} = 1.335$ mm for diameter 8.5 mm

The contact lens
The primary sag of the contact lens is

$x_L = s_1 + s_2 - s_3$ from Section 2.10

$s_1 = 0.818$ mm, $s_2 = 0.899$ mm, $s_3 = 0.601$ mm

∴ Primary sag $x_L = 1.116$ mm for diameter 8.5 mm

Axial edge clearance along 90

Axial edge clearance = TLT + $x_{90} - x_L$ from Section 4.3

$$= 0.01 + 1.335 - 1.116$$
$$= \underline{0.229 \text{ mm}}$$

(2) C2   7.7:7.00/10.50:8.50

Along 180

The cornea
As before

$r_0 = 7.90$ mm, $p = 0.8$

$x_{180} = 0.808$ mm for diameter 7 mm

The contact lens

$s_1 = 0.841$ mm for diameter 7 mm

TLT

TLT = $0.841 - 0.808$

$= 0.033$ mm

Thus the TLT has increased from 0.01 mm with BCOR 7.9 mm to 0.033 mm with BCOR 7.7 mm.

Along 90

The TLT is 0.033 mm.

The cornea
As before

$r_0 = 7.3$ mm, $p = 0.8$

$x_{90} = 1.335$ mm for diameter 8.5 mm

The contact lens

Primary sag $x_L = s_1 + s_2 - s_3$

$s_1 = 0.841$ mm, $s_2 = 0.899$ mm, $s_3 = 0.601$ mm

∴ Primary sag $x_L = 1.139$ mm for diameter 8.5 mm

Axial edge clearance along 90

Axial edge clearance $= TLT + x_{90} - x_L$

$= 0.033 + 1.335 - 1.139$

$= 0.229$ mm

This example illustrates that fitting steeper than alignment on the flatter meridian does not in fact theoretically reduce the edge standoff on the steeper meridian. It could be argued that this approach should be discouraged since it produces a lens which is flat on one meridian and steep on the other with no advantage as far as edge lift is concerned.

It will be instructive to repeat the example with an alternative lens design.

A cornea with vertex radii of 7.90 mm along 180 and 7.30 mm along 90 and a *p* value of 0.8 is fitted with a bicurve lens of the following specification:

C2 7.90:6.50/8.90:9.00

(1) What is the axial edge clearance along 90?
(2) What would the edge clearance be along 90 if the contact lens was changed to

C2 7.70:6.50/8.70:9.00

(1) C2 7.90:6.50/8.90:9.00 using *Figure 4.6*

Along 180

The cornea

$r_0 = 7.90$ mm $p = 0.8$

$$x_{180} = \frac{r_0}{p} - \sqrt{\left(\frac{r_0}{p}\right)^2 - \frac{y_1^2}{p}}$$

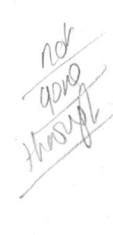

$x_{180} = 0.693$ mm for diameter 6.50 mm

The contact lens

Sag $s_1 = 0.699$ mm for diameter 6.5 mm

(using the sag equation in Section 2.10).

TLT

TLT = sag of contact lens s_1 − primary sag of cornea x_{180}
= 0.699 − 0.693 = 0.006 mm

Along 90
The TLT is 0.006 mm.

The cornea
$x_{90} = 1.512$ mm for diameter 9.00 mm

The contact lens

The primary sag of the contact lens is

$x_L = s_1 + s_2 - s_3$ from Section 2.10

See also *Figure 4.6*.

$s_1 = 0.699$ mm $s_2 = 1.221$ mm $s_3 = 0.614$ mm

∴ $x_L = 1.306$ mm for diameter 9.00 mm

Axial edge clearance

Axial edge clearance = TLT + $x_{90} - x_L$ from Section 4.3
= 0.006 + 1.512 − 1.306
= 0.212 mm

(2) C2 7.70:6.50/8.70:9.00

Along 180

The cornea
As before

$x_{180} = 0.693$ mm for diameter 6.50 mm

The contact lens

Sag $s_1 = 0.720$ mm for diameter 6.50 mm

TLT

TLT = 0.720 − 0.693 = 0.027 mm

Along 90
The TLT is 0.027 mm.

The cornea

As before

$x_{90} = 1.512$ mm for diameter 9.00 mm

The contact lens

Primary sag $x_L = s_1 + s_2 - s_3$

$s_1 = 0.720$ mm $s_2 = 1.254$ mm $s_3 = 0.630$ mm

∴ $x_L = 1.344$ mm for diameter 9.00 mm

Axial edge clearance
Axial edge clearance = TLT + $x_{90} - x_L$

$= 0.027 + 1.512 - 1.344$

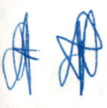

$= 0.195$ mm

Thus a change of lens design results in a reduction of axial edge clearance along the steeper corneal meridian when fitting steeper than alignment with the flat meridian. The astute reader will have realized that the first example resulted in the same edge clearance for both lenses because the BPOR was identical for the 7.9 mm and 7.7 mm central radii, and in both lenses the zone of contact with the cornea was the lens transition in the region of the flat corneal meridian. The steeper BCOR increased the TLT but the edge clearance was unaltered because the lens rests on the transition and the BPOR was identical in the two lenses. Thus lifting the apical region of the lens off the cornea will have no effect on the lens periphery when the lens rests on the transition. If the steeper lens possesses a BPOR which is also steeper, then the edge clearance decreases in both the flat and the steep meridians compared with that of the flatter lens.

4.9 Summary

- Corneal astigmatism is neutralized by a spherical back surface hard or GPH contact lens.
- Residual astigmatism is lenticular astigmatism.
- Back surface toric lenses induce astigmatism in the anterior fluid lens surface and this will require a front toric surface to compensate.
- A bitoric lens which corrects an eye with only corneal astigmatism can rotate without blurring the retinal image.
- Lenticular astigmatism requires a front surface toric and the lens must be rotationally stable.
- If a fitting set lens rotates in a clockwise direction then add this rotation to the standard notation of the cylinder axis found in the over-refraction, in order to relate the cylinder axis to the truncation or prism base–apex line.

5 Miscellaneous features

There are a number of topics which have not yet been covered that are not extensive enough to warrant a separate chapter. These topics are included in this chapter which therefore inevitably contains sections which have little or nothing in common with their neighbours. The chapter starts by considering the bifocal contact lens and continues with the correction of the aphakic eye. This is followed by a discussion of the galilean telescope, produced when a negative contact lens is combined with a positive spectacle lens to produce magnification for the visually disabled patient. The next section deals with contact lenses designed for use under water by the scuba diver. The optics of the soft lens is also included in this chapter, which could conceivably have been expected to require a full chapter of its own; however, much of what has already been discussed can be applied to the soft lens and the only novel feature is the lens flexibility. The final section deals with the deduction and calculation of radial lens thickness, which is not entirely unconnected to the soft lens since this calculation must be made in order to deduce the gas transmission through the contact lens.

5.1 Bifocal contact lenses

5.1.1 Front surface solid bifocals

Figure 5.1 illustrates the form of a front surface solid bifocal contact lens. The central area of the front surface consists of a curve of greater radius of curvature than that of the peripheral front surface. This results in a more positive power for the contact lens periphery. If the lens centres well on the eye when the primary position is adopted, then the central area can be used for distance vision. When the eye is depressed and converged in order to perform close work, then the visual axis of the eye is likely to pass through the more positive lens periphery. Let us suppose that a reading addition of +2.00 D is required for a particular eye and that the radius of curvature of the central area of the front surface is 8.45 mm; then

Bifocal contact lenses   107

Periphery used for near vision

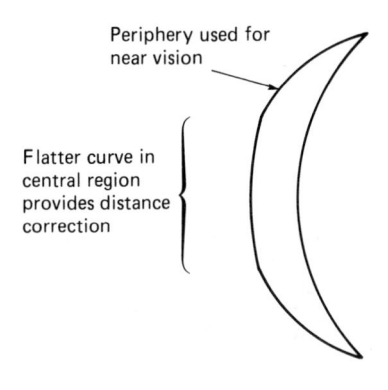

Flatter curve in central region provides distance correction

Figure 5.1. The front surface solid bifocal—the Wesley–Jessen design.

power of the central front surface $= \dfrac{490}{8.45}$ for a PMMA lens

$= +58.00$ D

and

power of the peripheral front surface $= +58.00 + 2.00$

$= +60.00$ D for a thin lens

∴ Radius of the peripheral front surface $= \dfrac{490}{60}$

$= 8.17$ mm for a thin lens

This assumes that paraxial theory can be applied to the lens periphery. We can take the lens thickness into consideration by applying the sag equation derived in Section 2.10 in order to deduce the central thickness that would have been present in the lens if the central flatter area was omitted.

In *Figure 5.2* BD represents the lens centre thickness. AD is the centre thickness that this lens would have if the central flatter curve was absent. It must therefore be considered as the centre thickness for the peripheral curve. If the lens central thickness BD is known then we need to find AB:

AB = AC − BC

If we take the front surface radii (as above) as 8.45 mm and 8.17 mm with a central area of diameter 5 mm and central lens thickness of 0.2 mm, then

$AC = 8.17 - \sqrt{8.17^2 - 2.5^2} = 0.392$ mm

108 Miscellaneous features

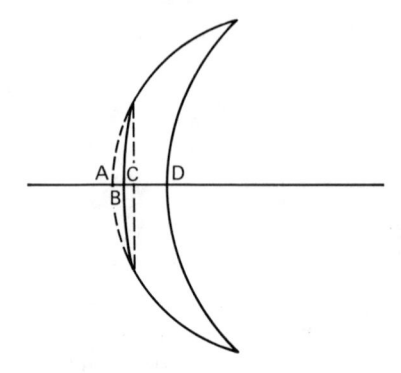

Figure 5.2. Centre thickness change in a bifocal contact lens. BD is the lens centre thickness; AD is the lens centre thickness for the peripheral curve; AB=AC−BC.

$$BC = 8.45 - \sqrt{8.45^2 - 2.5^2} = 0.378 \text{ mm}$$

$$\therefore AB = 0.014 \text{ mm}$$

Therefore, if BD is 0.2 mm, AD is 0.214 mm, the effective power of the central front surface at the back surface of the lens is

$$\frac{1000}{(1000/58) - (BD/n)} = +58.46 \text{ D}$$

The effective power of the peripheral front surface at the back surface of the lens is

$$\frac{1000}{(1000/60) - (AD/n)} = +60.52 \text{ D}$$

$$\therefore \text{Back vertex power of the addition} = +2.06 \text{ D}$$

We can conclude from this that, for typical PMMA corneal contact lens parameters, the effect of lens thickness can be ignored. There are, however, two significant problems associated with this type of bifocal. The first is that the small difference in radius of curvature between the two portions of the front surface makes this lens difficult to manufacture. The second is that tear fluid on the front surface of the lens may alter the power of the addition as shown in *Figure 5.3*, where the tear meniscus has formed between the contact lens and the lid margin when the eye is depressed for near work. Some practitioners therefore request a larger reading addition, and the extra positive power requested can be as high as 1.00 D. The greatest problem associated with this feature is that the effect is variable and dependent on the characteristics of the tears and the

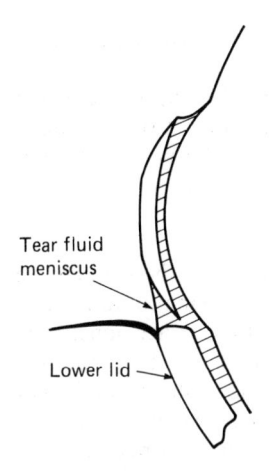

Figure 5.3. A fluid meniscus on the lens front surface reduces the power of the addition.

palpebral aperture, which makes prediction of an optimum addition unreliable.

An alternative approach is seen in *Figure 5.4* where the central area of the lens has the most positive power. In this design the lens is fitted to centre well at all positions of gaze. When the eye accommodates and converges for near, these changes will be accompanied by constriction of the pupil. It is likely in these circumstances that the pupil will be restricted mainly to the central area of the contact lens. In distance vision the larger pupil allows images to be formed by both the distance and near portions of the lens. The wearer must learn to ignore the out-of-focus image which arises from the central (near) portion in distance vision. The simultaneous presence of both the distance and near images has given rise to the term 'bivision bifocal'. The Williamson–Noble design is a bivision bifocal. The Wesley–Jessen design is described as an alternating bifocal. From a

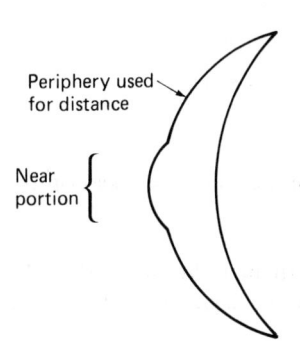

Figure 5.4. The Williamson–Noble bifocal design.

practical point of view there will probably be a bivision element in an alternating bifocal.

The problems of manufacturing the lens and the requirement of a higher reading addition due to tear meniscus formation are much the same for the Williamson–Noble design as for the Wesley–Jessen.

5.1.2 Back surface solid bifocals

An alternative to the front surface bifocal is to work the segment on the back surface of the lens. This design is easier to manufacture due to the fact that, when in position on the eye, the surface generating the segment is in contact with fluid and not with air. Therefore the difference in radius of curvature between the distance and near portions required to achieve the addition is considerably greater than with front surface bifocals, making the manufacture of the lens a less daunting proposition. The back surface solid bifocal is an alternating design. *Figure 5.5.* illustrates the form of a typical back surface design. It is immediately apparent that the segment is providing the distance vision.

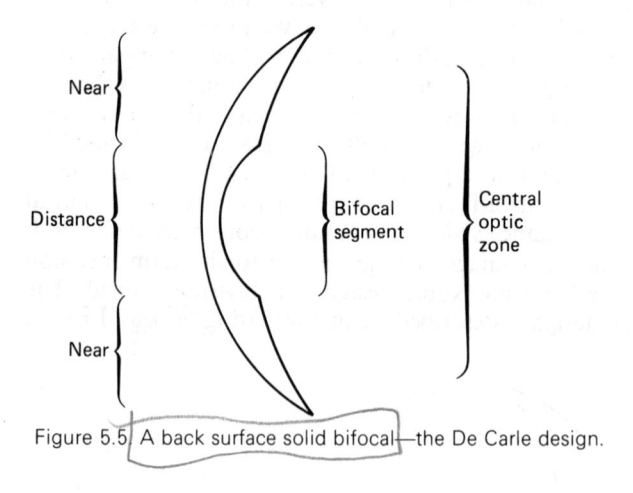

Figure 5.5. A back surface solid bifocal—the De Carle design.

Let us take a typical example. The distance lens specification is

C2   7.90:7.00/8.90:9.00 BVP −5.00 D

We require a back surface solid bifocal with an addition of +3.00 D. What radius of curvature is required for the segment? What is the power of the addition in air?

Bifocal contact lenses 111

The distance BVP is of no direct consequence in this problem. We need to know the power of the back surface on the eye.

On the eye
The power on the eye of a surface of radius 7.9 mm is

$$\frac{(1336-1490)}{7.9} = -19.49 \text{ D}$$

Since we need a +3.00 D addition, the bifocal segment must be more negative by 3.00 D.

∴ Power of bifocal segment surface on the eye = −22.49 D

∴ Radius of curvature of this surface = $\frac{(1336-1490)}{-22.49}$ = 6.85 mm

In air
Power of surface of radius 7.9 mm in air = $\frac{490}{7.9}$ = −62.03 D

Power of surface of radius 6.85 mm in air = $\frac{490}{6.85}$ = −71.53 D

∴ Power of the addition in air = +9.50 D

The large difference in the two powers makes lens checking easier than with the front surface solid bifocals. We have, in this treatment, ignored the fact that the back vertex of the distance and near curves do not exactly coincide but, as we have already seen, this does not influence the answer in any significant way. If we considered the bifocal segment diameter in our example to be 5 mm, then the back vertex position will differ by 0.0665 mm between the distance and reading surfaces. This shift of position will produce a 0.34 D error in the lens power in air. The central back surface is worked deeper into the lens, which results in its effective negative power at the back vertex of the reading surface being 0.34 D less negative. However, it must also be noted that because this central curve reduces the lens thickness the light incident on its surface will possess slightly less positive vergence (around 0.2 D) which is a compensating influence. When the lens is on the eye the 0.34 D error is reduced to 0.03 D.

We can deduce from the above that the power of the addition in air will be approximately three times that on the eye. When checking these lenses the power of the addition in air will have to be calculated; this can be simplified to the relationship derived below.

The power of the back surface of the contact lens in air is

$$F_2 = \frac{1-n_p}{r_2}$$

where n_p is the refractive index of the contact lens. If this lens is placed on the eye then the back surface interfaces with the tears and the back surface power is reduced. F_2 becomes $(n_t - n_p)/r_2$ where n_t is the refractive index of the tears.

$$\text{Ratio of these two powers} = \frac{1-n_p}{n_t - n_p}$$

$$= \frac{n_p - 1}{n_p - n_t}$$

$$\therefore \text{Power of add in air} = \frac{n_p - 1}{n_p - n_t} A$$

where A is the power of the add required on the eye. If we take n_p as 1.490 and n_t as 1.336, the relationship reduces to

power of add in air = 3.18 × power of add required on the eye

This relationship also holds good for the cylindrical power of a toric back surface.

5.1.3 Fused bifocals

The fused bifocal is an alternating design which has the appearance of a spectacle bifocal lens in that the segment is a D, B or crescent shape positioned in the lower part of the lens, with the segment material possessing a higher refractive index than that of the main lens.

Figure 5.6 illustrates the form of the fused bifocal. The manufacturer must calculate the radius of curvature of the depression curve, i.e. the curve of the interface between the segment and the main lens.

Let us take an example. The distance specification of the contact lens is

C2   7.90:7.00/8.90:9.00 BVP −5.00 D

We require a fused bifocal with an addition of +3.00 D. What is the radius of curvature of the depression curve? What is the power of the contact lens in air? Assume the refractive index of the main lens is 1.490 with the refractive index of the segment being 1.560.

Bifocal contact lenses 113

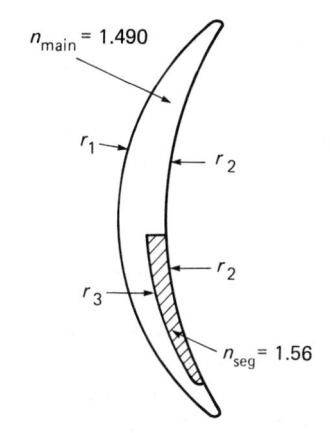

Figure 5.6. The fused bifocal.

The distance BVP is of no direct consequence in this problem.

On the eye

Power of the lower surface of
radius 7.90 mm
$$= \frac{(1336-1560)}{7.9} = -28.35 \text{ D}$$

Power of the upper surface of
radius 7.90 mm
$$= \frac{(1336-1490)}{7.9} = -19.49 \text{ D}$$

Difference $\qquad = 8.86 \text{ D}$

Thus, the back surface power of the lower part of the lens is 8.86 D more negative than the upper part, and we require this section of the lens to be 3.00 D more positive than the upper part. Therefore the power of the bifocal contact surface must be $+8.86+3.00 = +11.86$ D to compensate and give the addition requested.

$$\therefore r_3 = \frac{(1560-1490)}{+11.86} = 5.90 \text{ mm}$$

N.B. The segment has been assumed to be thin.

In air
The difference between this lens and the back surface solid bifocal is that, for the fused bifocal, the back surface curve r_2 is the same for both the distance and near portions. Therefore the power of the fluid

lens is the same for both distance and near. If we consider the back surface powers in air:

Power of the upper surface of
radius 7.90 mm $= \dfrac{-490}{7.9} = -62.03\,\text{D}$

Power of the lower surface of
radius 7.90 mm $= \dfrac{-560}{7.9} = -70.89\,\text{D}$

Therefore the back surface power of the lower part of the lens is 8.86 D more negative than the upper part. This is exactly the same power difference as that found on the eye. Thus the power difference between distance and near portions is constant. We can therefore see that the power of the add on the eye is the same as the power of the add in air for this type of bifocal.

The segment is usually shaped something like an ophthalmic spectacle bifocal lens D segment. This means that the contact lens must be rotationally stable in order to maintain a correct position on the eye, and this is usually achieved by prism ballasting. The segment shape ensures that the optical centre of the segment is very close to the segment top. There is therefore little or no jump at the segment top in this design. The curved top of the crescent-shaped segment helps to maintain an acceptable performance even if the lens orientation varies.

5.2 The correction of the aphakic eye

The aphakic eye usually requires a substantial positive power (often around +12.00 D) to effect a correction. This means that a measurement of vertex distance is essential during the refraction and a contact lens made to correct an individual eye will be more powerful than the spectacle correction. The spectacle correction, however, will suffer from a number of disadvantages.

5.2.1 The motor field of view or field of fixation

In *Figure 5.7* we see an eye which has rotated to look through the upper extremity A of a spectacle lens whose optical centre is at S. This illustrates the extent of the field constriction. Also any object positioned in the shaded areas of *Figure 5.7* would not be seen at all since this type of correction results in a ring scotoma arising out of

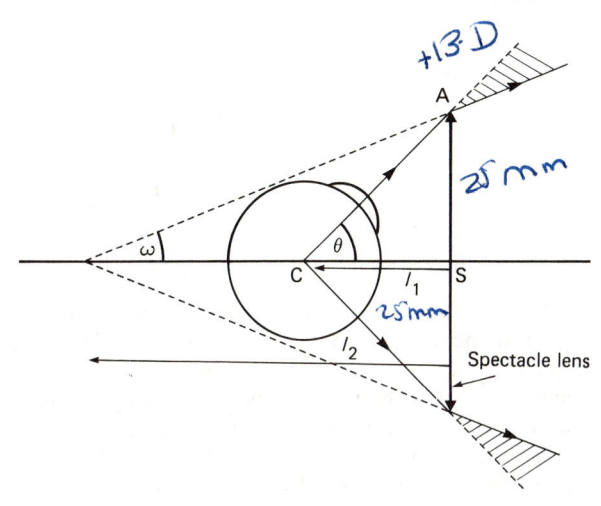

Figure 5.7. The motor field or field of fixation. C is the centre of rotation of the eye.

the prismatic deviation produced at the lens periphery. This appears to cause most distress to the wearer when observing at intermediate distances around 1–3 m.

The deviation of the limiting light ray at A can be calculated by regarding the centre of rotation of the eye as a point object. Let us assume that the lens diameter is 50 mm and the distance CS is 25 mm.

Lens semi-diameter = 25 mm

$\therefore \tan \theta = \dfrac{25}{25}$ and $\theta = 45°$

$\therefore$ Field of fixation without the spectacle lens = 90°

Field of fixation with the spectacle lens in place = 2ω

In order to deduce ω we must first know l_2. Let us suppose that the lens has a power of +13.00 D.

Object vergence $L_1 = \dfrac{1000}{-25}$ = −40.00 D

Lens power = +13.00 D

$\therefore$ Image vergence L_2 = −27.00 D

$$\therefore l_2 = \frac{1000}{-27} = -37.04 \text{ mm}$$

$$\tan \omega = \frac{25}{37.04} = 0.675$$

$$\therefore \omega = 34° 1'$$

$$\therefore \text{Field of fixation for the corrected aphakic} = 2\omega = 68° 2'$$

It is as well to remember that the spectacle lens will suffer from oblique aberrations and the visual acuity may show some deterioration when the visual axis passes through the spectacle lens periphery. Also the spectacle lens may cause distortion of the retinal image, which some patients find difficult to adapt to. The spectacle lens may need constant adjustment to maintain the desired vertex distance. However, the 'Jack in the box' effect causes major adaptive problems.

5.2.2 The Jack in the box effect

If an aphakic eye, corrected by a spectacle lens, is in the primary position, it may be aware of an object, let us say, to the right of fixation. If the eye in question turns to the right to look at this object then the pupil will be displaced laterally to the right during the rotation, and this displacement may be enough for the object to disappear into the ring scotoma. As a result of this phenomenon, the wearer sees objects that are eccentric to central fixation disappearing when he or she attempts to fixate the object of interest, only to find the object reappearing when central fixation is resumed. The patient must become accustomed to rotating the head instead of rotating the eyes in order to deal with this problem.

5.2.3 Retinal image size

The topic of retinal image size, spectacle magnification and relative spectacle magnification was discussed in Chapter 1. The summary here is derived from the relationships described in that chapter (Section 1.5 and Section 1.6).

The high plus spectacle lens will produce a magnification of the retinal image size which increases with increased vertex distance. The retinal image size will typically be around 25% larger in a corrected aphakic than in an emmetrope. A contact lens correction results in the correcting lens being very near the entrance pupil of the eye and the spectacle magnification is much reduced; however, it is not unity and it is increased by an increase in the shape factor (see Section 1.5) of the correcting lens. An examination of typical contact lens shape factors reveals that scleral lenses have larger shape factors than corneal or soft lenses. Therefore a scleral lens produces a larger retinal image because of its larger shape factor, which is due in the main to a larger central thickness than that which occurs in the corneal or soft lens. This is particularly noteworthy in the case of the monocular aphakic who cannot possibly fuse the two retinal images when a spectacle correction is used. The contact lens correction should be one which limits the retinal image size as much as possible. Therefore, in this respect at least, the corneal or soft lens is preferable to the scleral lens. However, even so, the lens will produce a small magnification of the corrected retinal image and, although the monocular aphakic may well be able to fuse the two images, some aniseikonic adaptive problems are to be expected. Many aphakic contact lens wearers require auxiliary spectacles and this is quite likely in a monocular aphakic who needs a prescription for the other eye. In this case you can over-correct the plus (or give a contact lens sighted for reading): the negative distance spectacle lens will reduce the retinal image size, though the combination you need to equalize retinal image sizes may not give you an ideal reading add in the contact lens.

5.2.4 Near vision

The aphakic eye is incapable of accommodating in order to focus near work. Some practitioners have suggested adding extra positive power to the distance correction in order to help the aphakic with intermediate and near work. However, there appear to be some reservations, and caution on the part of the practitioner is advised. Stone and Francis (1980) have noted that the positive spherical aberration in a high plus contact lens produces a correction which may well be around 2.00 D more positive in the lens periphery than at its centre. Thus an aphakic whose contact lenses ride high when the eyes are depressed for close work may well be able to manage without a supplementary reading correction. If, on the other hand, some extra positive power is needed for close work this may most conveniently be prescribed as a pair of reading spectacles which contain the reading addition to be used in conjunction with the distance contact lenses.

5.2.5 Lenticular lenses

A contact lens with a high positive power will possess a centre of

118 Miscellaneous features

gravity which is well forward, and this encourages a corneal lens to drop into a low riding position on the eye. Some improvement in position may be attained by reducing the central thickness of the lens, which usually means that the lens must be made in lenticular form as illustrated in *Figure 5.8*. This illustrates the point that the carrier zone (i.e. the lens periphery) should display a slightly increasing thickness with eccentricity in order to encourage the upper lid to hold the lens in a more central position. The axial thickness of the junction should not be less than about 0.14 mm. The calculations involved in determining the lens parameters are illustrated in the following example.

A corneal lens of the following specification

C2 7.80:6.00/8.80:9.00 BVP +12.00 D
central thickness 0.26 mm

is to be made up in lenticular form with an FCOD of 6 mm and an FPOR of 10 mm. What is the axial lens thickness at the junction of the front surface curves? What is the edge thickness?

In this example the FCOD equals the BCOD, which will allow a minimum centre thickness without encroaching into the central optic region of the lens. This probably represents the best compromise. However, some practitioners advise an FCOD larger than the BCOD.

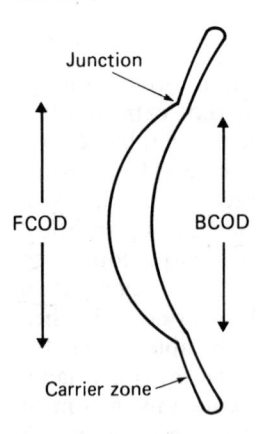

Figure 5.8. A lenticulated high plus contact lens.

From *Figure 5.9* we see that

$$t_j = t_c + s_b - s_f$$

We have been given a BCOR of 7.80 mm, a lens centre thickness of 0.26 mm, and a BVP of +12.00 D.

This allows us to calculate the central front surface radius which is found to be 6.635 mm.

We can now use the sag equation

$$s = r - \sqrt{r^2 - y^2}$$

to calculate s_f and s_b:

$s_f = 6.635 - \sqrt{6.635^2 - 3^2} = 0.717$ mm

$s_b = 7.80 - \sqrt{7.80^2 - 3^2} = 0.6$ mm

$t_c = 0.26$ mm

$\therefore\ t_j = 0.26 + 0.6 - 0.717$

$t_j = 0.143$ mm

We now know the thickness of the lens at the junction and we can use this to proceed to the edge thickness. In *Figure 5.10*

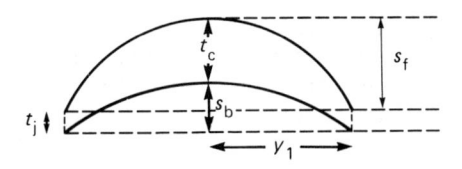

Figure 5.9. The central contact lens in cross section. t_j is the axial thickness at the junction.

$t_e = (s_1 - s_2) + t_j - (s_3 - s_4)$

$s_1 = 8.8 - \sqrt{8.8^2 - 4.5^2} = 1.238$ mm

$s_2 = 8.8 - \sqrt{8.8^2 - 3^2} = 0.527$ mm

$s_1 - s_2 = 0.711$ mm

$s_3 = 10 - \sqrt{10^2 - 4.5^2} = 1.07$ mm

$s_4 = 10 - \sqrt{10^2 - 3^2} = 0.461$ mm

$s_3 - s_4 = 0.609$ mm

120 Miscellaneous features

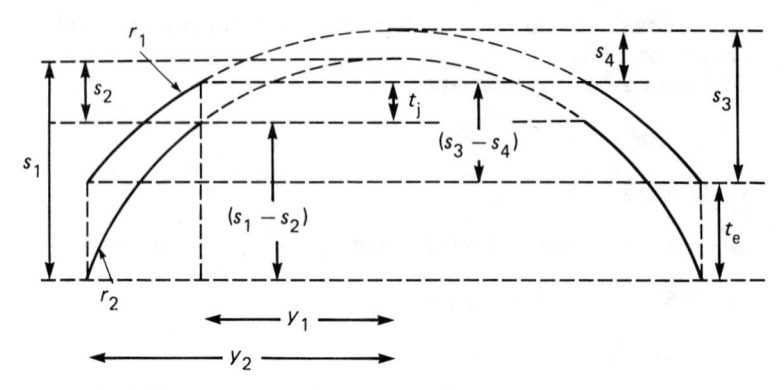

Figure 5.10. The carrier zone of the contact lens.

$$\therefore t_e = 0.711 + 0.143 - 0.609$$

$$t_e = 0.245 \text{ mm}$$

In clinical practice the practitioner needs to adopt an iterative technique where likely lens parameters are substituted in order to calculate the thicknesses, with the calculations repeated until acceptable thicknesses are achieved. This process is much more attractive if a computer is used to repeat the calculations. A computer program is included in Chapter 7 for this very purpose.

5.3 The low vision aid telescope

The galilean telescope is used as a spectacle-mounted magnification device for the visually disabled requiring help for distance, intermediate or near work. The distance system is illustrated in *Figure 5.11*, where a distant object h subtends a visual angle ω at the telescope objective lens O which is separated from the eyepiece lens E by distance d. The diagram illustrates that the incident pencil of light rays coming from the top of the object emerges from the eyepiece still as a parallel pencil but one which reveals a visual angle of ω'. *Figure 5.11.* also illustrates that, for a telescope set for distance viewing, the principal focii F_1' and F_2' coincide. The light rays from the distant point source (the upper point of the object) would be focussed in the plane F_1' if the eyepiece were removed. Thus the light incident on the eyepiece is converging on to its principal focus F_2 and this ensures that the light emerges as a parallel pencil.

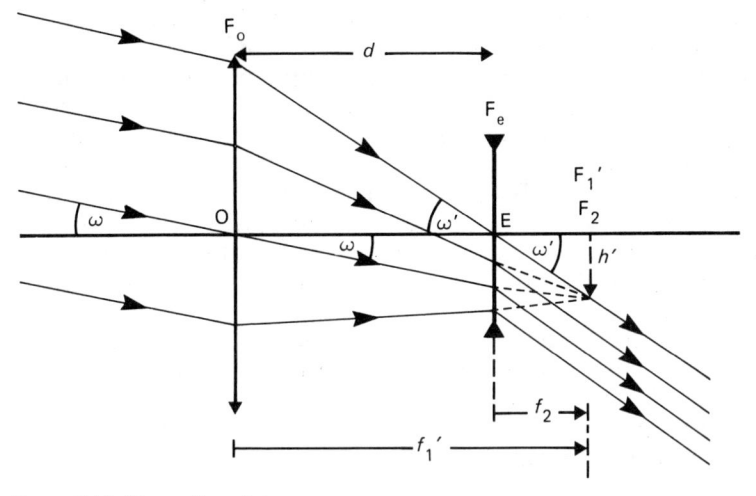

Figure 5.11. The galilean telescope.

The magnification can be defined as the ratio of the visual angle of the object ω to the visual angle seen through the telescope ω'.

$$\therefore \text{Magnification} = \omega'/\omega$$

$$\tan \omega = \frac{h'}{f_1'} \qquad \tan \omega' = \frac{h'}{f_2}$$

$$\therefore \text{Magnification} = \frac{h'/f_2}{h'/f_1'} = \frac{f_1'}{f_2} = \frac{F_E}{F_O}$$

where F_E is the dioptric power of the eyepiece (ignoring its sign) and F_O is the dioptric power of the objective when f_1' and f_2 are measured in metres.

$$\therefore \text{Magnification} = \frac{\text{power of eyepiece}}{\text{power of objective}}$$

Also

$$f_2 = f_1' - d$$

$$\text{Magnification} = \frac{f_1'}{f_2} = \frac{f_1'}{f_1' - d}$$

$$\text{Magnification} = \frac{1}{(1 - d/f_1')} = \frac{1}{(1 - dF_O)}$$

where F_o is again the dioptric power of the objective and d is the separation between the objective and eyepiece in metres.

The cosmetic appearance of a conventional telescope can be dramatically improved if it is made up by using a positive spectacle lens as the objective and a negative contact lens as the eyepiece. This initially attractive idea, however, rapidly becomes less attractive when consideration is given to the fact that the lens separation d will be the vertex distance of the spectacles and must inevitably therefore be small. This means that the lens powers must be large, and even then the magnification achieved will be modest. Let us take a typical example.

A $+25.00$ D spectacle lens is to be glazed into a spectacle frame of vertex distance 14 mm. What power is required for a contact lens to act as the eyepiece for a galilean telescope, assuming the eye is emmetropic and requires to view distant objects? What magnification will be produced by this device?

In *Figure 5.12*,

power of the objective	$= +25.00$ D
$\therefore f_1'$	$= 40$ mm
d	$= 14$ mm
$\therefore f_2$	$= 26$ mm
$\therefore$ Power of the eyepiece	$= 38.46$ D

$$\text{Magnification} = \frac{\text{power of eyepiece}}{\text{power of objective}}$$

$$= \frac{38.46}{25} = 1.54 \times$$

The problems become immediately obvious. The high plus spectacle lens will not be particularly good from a cosmetic point of view. The high minus contact lens will be difficult to fit and may never be particularly comfortable. Any movement of the contact lens will produce apparent movement of the visual field since the contact lens is now the eyepiece of a telescope. Finally, as with all galilean telescopes, the field of view will be significantly restricted.

5.3.1 Field of view

Strictly speaking, we must be most concerned with the field of

The LVA telescope

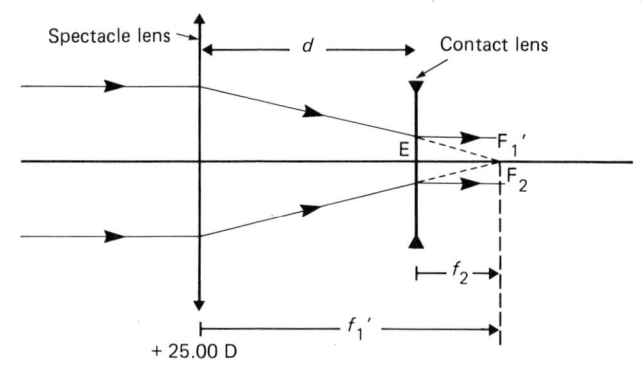

Figure 5.12. The contact lens/spectacle lens telescope.

fixation. We simply need to trace a limiting light ray from the centre of rotation of the eye in order to determine the angle of emergence from the objective lens.

The light ray in *Figure 5.13* is a limiting light ray that goes to C, the centre of rotation of the eye. If we assume that the distance from C to the contact lens is 13 mm and we also assume that we are dealing with the telescopic system of the previous example, then $d = 14$ mm. Let us also assume that the objective diameter is 32 mm, i.e. $y = 16$ mm.

$$\tan \theta = \frac{16}{13 + 14} = 0.5926$$

Figure 5.13. The field of fixation for a contact lens telescope. The contact lens is assumed to maintain a well centred position on the cornea. C is the centre of rotation of the eye. 2ω is the field of fixation.

The eye needs to rotate $2\theta = 61° 18'$ in order to look from edge to edge of the field of fixation.

Object distance $CO = -27$ mm

giving an object vergence of

$\dfrac{1000}{-27}$ = -37.04 D

Objective power F_o = $+25.00$ D

∴ Image vergence = -12.04 D

∴ Distance $C_2'O = \dfrac{1000}{-12.04} = -83.06$ mm

$\tan \omega = \dfrac{16}{83.06} = 0.1926$

$\omega = 10.9°$

Field of fixation $2\omega = 21° 48'$

5.3.2 The Telecon system

Figure 5.14 illustrates the Telecon system introduced by Filderman. The contact lens has a central circular zone of diameter 2.5 mm which is sighted BVP -50.00 D. The objective is mounted at a

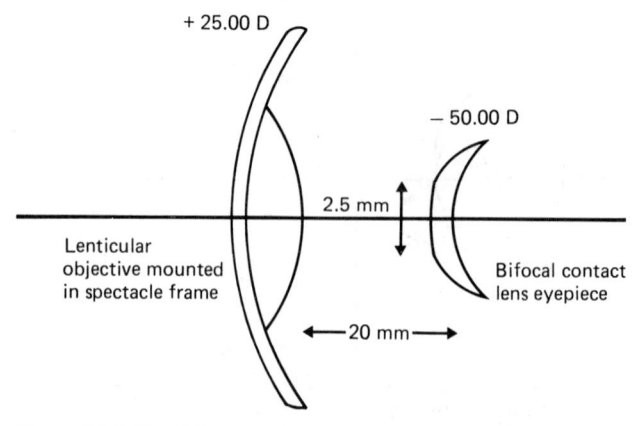

Figure 5.14. The Telecon system.

vertex distance of 20 mm, and consists of a plano-meniscus carrier with a +25.00 D lenticular aperture cemented onto the carrier. This provides a system which allows for image magnification using the central zone of the contact lens and the spectacle lenticular, with the advantage of also observing an unmagnified periphery via the contact lens peripheral zone (which can carry the distance correction) and the plano-periphery of the spectacle lenticular. The magnification achieved with this system is 2 ×.

However, once again the practical problems encountered in fitting and adapting to this system are considerable.

Bennett (1985) has described the effects of wearing a contact lens telescope which produced nausea after a short time. Chromatic aberration, pincushion distortion and apparent movement of the visual field all produced noticeable effects with the magnification, making estimation of distance very difficult.

5.3.3 Near vision

A distance telescope is most conveniently converted to a near telescope by using a positive-powered lens placed in front of the objective. A +4.00 D lens, for example, would convert the divergent light rays from an object 25 cm away to a parallel pencil, which the distance telescope is designed to deal with. In the case of the Telecon system, a second reduced aperture lens bonded to the lower section of the carrier portion, with a power which is 4.00 D more positive than the central reduced aperture lens, provides magnification for near if required.

5.4 Underwater lenses

There are two basic approaches to correction of vision under water. The first is to equip the scuba diver with a scleral lens on which is mounted an air cell. This is in effect a miniaturized face mask. The second approach consists of manufacturing a bifocal scleral lens which is sighted with one power for surface vision and the other for underwater vision.

5.4.1 The air cell lens

Figure 5.15 illustrates a typical air cell design. The flat plate and air cell ensure that light is travelling in air before being refracted by the contact lens optic. The lens therefore performs in exactly the same way as a conventional face mask. The flat plate is angled as shown in

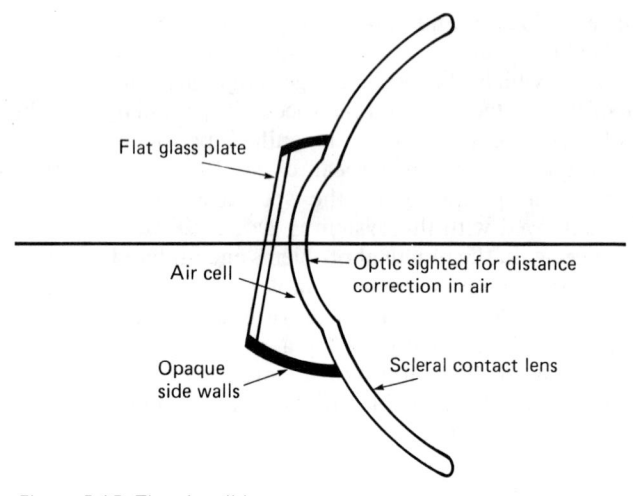

Figure 5.15. The air cell lens.

order to help make upper lid movements more comfortable and derive more lens support from the lower lid.

The wearer sees everything at the apparent distance under water, owing to refraction at the flat plate. The opaque side walls restrict the field of vision (but not the field of fixation). The field of view is further reduced under water by refraction at the flat plate. The plate angle must be very similar in the two eyes if diplopia is to be avoided under water. If either lens rides lower or higher than its fellow, then this will induce vertical diplopia under water. The air in the air cell must be absolutely dry if internal condensation is to be avoided. The air cell may collapse or leak at depth where the water pressure increases (the pressure increases by one atmosphere for every 10 m of depth).

5.4.2 The bifocal lens

This was originally suggested by Bennett (1965). *Figure 5.16* illustrates the Douthwaite design (1971) which is fitted in order to discourage lens lag. The low levels of light under water allow the large pupil to utilize the peripheral area of the flint glass button which is bonded to the scleral lens with an epoxy resin. The higher light levels on the surface produce pupil constriction which allows the central section of the button to dominate the image formation. This design is free of the disadvantages listed for the air cell lens. The

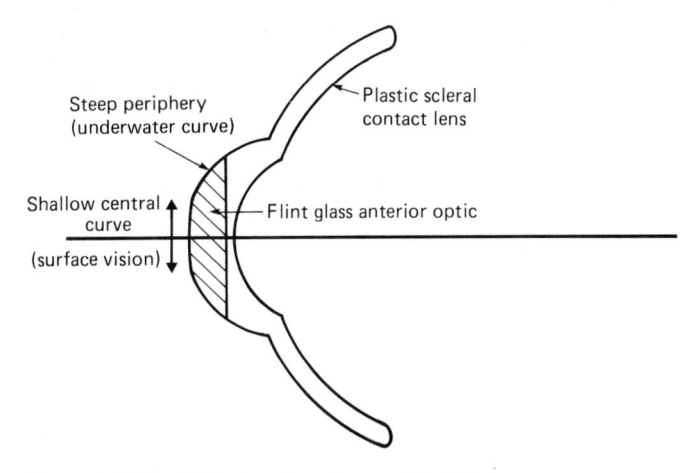

Figure 5.16. The bifocal underwater contact lens.

front surface radii of the flint glass button are easily calculated following the recommendations of Section 5.1. The design might be further improved by moving the shallow curve zone into the lower half of the flint button, since divers under water tend to look up towards their foreheads as they swim horizontally face downward and yet on the surface they tread water in a vertical position with their heads well back which results in their looking down their noses in order to scan the horizon.

5.5 Soft lenses

The flexibility of the soft contact lens inevitably means that optical calculations or calculations concerning the lens specification are open to question. It has already been noted, for example, that the fluid lens formed behind a soft contact lens on the eye is likely to have a power around plano to -0.50 D; however, this cannot be reliably predicted and the changes occurring in the fluid lens power when the central optic radius is changed again are not predictable.

The method of manufacture is to cut, spin cast, or mould the lens in a dry form. This can be done with precision but the material must then be hydrated which will alter the physical parameters of the lens. The manufacturer must assume a particular swell factor and produce a dry lens which on hydration will swell to the desired specification. If a swell factor of 60% is assumed then the manufacturer expects the lens parameters to increase by 60%. The actual swell factor achieved may vary from the assumed value and this is why the precision of soft lens manufacture is not as high as that of the hard and GP lens.

5.5.1 Power changes of soft lenses

If a soft lens is placed on a particular eye it may well warp so that the back surface takes up the curvature of the cornea on which it rests. This is called lens flexure. In these circumstances the front surface radius will also alter and these induced changes may well affect the power of the contact lens. In order to investigate the consequence of power changes due to the lens bending on the eye we must make some assumptions about induced changes in the lens parameters. Strachan (1973) claims that the 'wrap factor' remains constant. If a lens of back optic radius 9 mm is fitted to a cornea of 8 mm radius, the wrap factor is 9/8 which equals 1.125. Thus the new front surface radius is the old front surface radius divided by 1.125. Baron (1975) suggested that a change in back surface radius will be accompanied by an almost equal change in the front surface radius. The most useful work on this subject was published by Bennett (1976) who assumed that the lens volume remains unchanged; there is no redistribution of lens thickness; with the lens front surface remaining spherical when resting on a spherical cornea. He deduced tables for both positive and negative lenses which lead to the conclusion that the power change induced by flexure is independent of the initial power of the lens. The power changes are greatest for thick lenses and steep radii. As the lens steepens, its power becomes more negative. The fundamental principle is illustrated in *Figure 5.17*

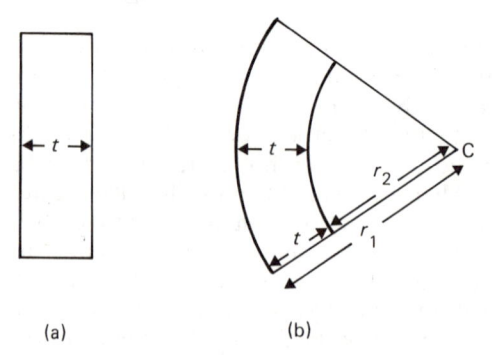

Figure 5.17. (a) A flat parallel plate, (b) bent to form a concentric meniscus lens. C is the centre of curvature of both surfaces.

where a flat parallel plate is bent into a concentric meniscus lens. In these circumstances $r_1 = r_2 + t$ where r_1 is the radius of curvature of the front surface and r_2 is the radius of curvature of the back surface with t representing the radial thickness of the plate. It will be recalled that for an afocal thick lens

$$r_1 = r_2 + \frac{n-1}{n} t$$

(see Section 2.3). This means that the concentric lens has a front surface radius which is too long to maintain the afocal nature of the flat plate. This excessive radius produces insufficient positive power for the front surface which results in a negative back vertex power. Thus, bending a lens to reduce the radii of curvature induces increasing negative power and the effect is more pronounced with thicker lenses. Bennett's investigation included powered lenses where the same changes were found to occur. He derived an equation to quantify the changes:

$$\Delta F_V' = -300t \left(\frac{1}{r_2'^2} - \frac{1}{r_2^2} \right)$$

for a lens refractive index of 1.44, where $\Delta F_V'$ is the change in BVP, t is the centre thickness, r_2 is the original back surface radius and r_2' is the new back surface radius after bending the lens.

If we substitute typical values in the above equation we can get some idea of the degree of power change.

If

$t = 0.3$ mm, $r_2 = 8$ mm, $r_2' = 7$ mm

then

$\Delta F_V' = -300 \times 0.3 \, (0.0204 - 0.0156)$

$= -0.43$ D

The equation was found to be in close agreement with that derived by Wichterle (1967) by an entirely different route. We can therefore conclude that steepening a soft lens will induce an increase of negative power, owing to the flexure of the lens, and this increase is independent of the contact lens BVP but is greater for thick lenses than for thin.

If a spherical lens is fitted to a toric cornea, the the lens steepening on the steeper corneal meridian will induce some negative power increase which will help to correct the corneal astigmatism. It must be remembered that the soft lens may not distort to the full corneal toricity but the lens material is of higher refractive index than that of the cornea. It may therefore transmit all or almost all of the corneal astigmatism at the lens front surface. However, it must also be pointed out that the vergence change at the contact lens back surface/anterior fluid lens surface interface will provide some partial correction of this astigmatism which is also influenced by the contact lens refractive index. The power change in air described by Bennett does not take into account the power change induced at the anterior surface of the fluid lens. If the lens steepens on the eye, then the small negative power increase is much less than the positive power increase of the fluid lens (this would be +6.00 D for a radius change from 8 to 7 mm), which results in most of the astigmatism being transmitted through the lens.

The flexure may be of further consequence when performing a fitting with an over-refraction check. If, for example, a 7.9 mm radius lens was resting on a cornea without any flexure and the over-refraction suggested a BVP reuired of −2.00 D, and this lens was removed and replaced by a lens of radius 8.1 mm, the new lens will presumably steepen on the eye so that the fluid lens power remains unchanged; however, the lens itself will have become more negative.

During the time that a soft lens is worn, the lens temperature will increase from room to body temperature and this will encourage the lens to steepen. Also evaporation from the front surface of the lens will increase the refractive index of the lens material and again encourages the lens towards steepening. In the case of a negatively powered lens the refractive index increase leads to a more negative lens power. The partial dehydration, however, may increase the lens rigidity which will reduce the tendency towards flexure.

Thus there are a number of interrelated factors which influence the final outcome of the power of the correction.

5.5.2 Soft lenses and astigmatism

The general recommendation for soft lenses is that if the ocular astigmatism is over 0.75 D then the visual acuity may be unacceptably low or variable with spherical lenses. This recommendation applies to astigmatism where the principal meridians are near horizontal and near vertical. If the principal meridians are oblique then the astigmatic tolerance may have to be lowered to less than 0.50 D. If the lens is a thicker or lower water content lens then it may transmit less of the corneal astigmatism, although this point is disputed. Conversely a thinner or higher water content lens may well transmit all the corneal astigmatism as a result of the lens warping into a toric form to match the corneal toricity. In the case of a thin lens the flexure will be less likely to cause an increase in negative power as the lens steepens on the steep corneal meridian. As with hard and GPH lenses, any lenticular astigmatism will still be present in its entirety. An astigmatic correction can be effected by using soft toric contact lenses.

5.5.2.1 Back surface torics

The typical back surface toric fitting set consists of a series of spherical lenses, usually with a truncation, which allows an assessment of the lens orientation to be made. The lenses may also have a prism worked into them to aid the rotational stability. If such a lens is fitted to a toric cornea it will warp into a toric form and transmit most of the corneal astigmatism, because the front contact lens surface takes up a toric form with the back toric surface partially neutralized by the fluid lens anterior surface.

Let us suppose that the patient's keratometry readings are

8.30 along 5/7.70 along 95

with a spectacle correction of

-6.50 DS$/-4.00$ DC $\times$ 5 at a vertex distance of 12 mm

This gives a refraction of -6.00 DS$/-3.25$ DC $\times$ 5 at the cornea rounded to the nearest 0.25 D.

Let us suppose that the best fitting lens from the fitting set is marked with a radius of 8.60 mm. It is assumed that the 8.60 mm radius curve will produce a near afocal fluid lens along the flatter corneal meridian which has an error of -6.00 D. The steeper meridian, being more myopic, will require extra negative power. In our example the steeper corneal meridian requires an extra negative power of -3.25 D.

The power of the back surface along the 5 meridian is

$$\frac{1-n}{r} = \frac{-444}{8.6} = -51.63 \text{ D}$$

The 95 meridian must be 3.25 D more negative, so its power must be -54.88 D. Therefore the radius of the 95 meridian must be

$$\frac{-444}{-54.88} = 8.09 \text{ mm}$$

If we use a back surface radius of 8.09 mm along 95 then this results in a contact lens with 3.25 D more negative power, which corrects the astigmatism.

These recommendations make the assumption that the fluid lens has the same power (approximately afocal) for both meridians, which will only be the case if the lens back surface approximates to the corneal curvature. If we then picture the contact lens, tear lens, and cornea all separated by thin air films we can see that the corneal astigmatism has been neutralized (see *Figure 5.18*).

In *Figure 5.18* the back surface of the contact lens must be overcorrecting the corneal astigmatism; however, if the fluid lens is to be approximately afocal in both meridians, the toric back surface lens will warp on the eye, so that both surface curvatures in the vertical meridian will steepen. This inevitably means that the front surface power of the contact lens will be more positive than the front surface power with the lens in its non-deformed state along the vertical meridian and this extra positive power will neutralize the back surface over-correction of the corneal astigmatism. It is therefore obvious from the above that although the lens is manufactured with a toric back surface and a spherical front surface it will in fact, on the eye, possess two toric surfaces. An alternative approach to clarify the picture is to note that the back surface toric lens on the eye will possess a front surface which is toric with the front surface toricity being less than is the case with spherical lenses. In our example the toric lens back surface vertical meridian will warp 3.25 D less than a spherical lens, which implies that the vertical meridian of the lens front surface will be approximately 3.25 D less

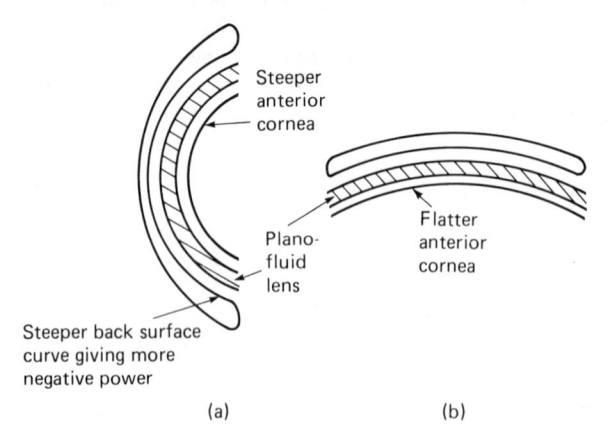

Figure 5.18. The soft contact lens/fluid lens/anterior cornea system separated by thin air films (a) along 95 and (b) along 5.

positive than is the case with a spherical lens. Thus the toric lens has a front surface power which is 3.25 D more negative in the vertical meridian, and the lens therefore corrects the astigmatism. The above assumes thin lens theory which results in no power change induced by flexure and therefore maintenance of the BVP as the lens curvatures steepen on the eye.

Ideally the truncation should take up a horizontal orientation in which case the lens order will be as follows:

8.60/8.10 −6.00 13.00 T5

(the 8.1 mm radius being the nearest approximation to the 8.09 mm found by calculation).

If the truncation rotates clockwise then this rotation must be added to the axis orientation of the prescription to compensate.

Let us suppose that the truncation orientation is 170 (which is a 10° clockwise rotation). The lens order would then be as follows:

8.60/8.10 −6.00 13.00 T15

That is, the flat meridian must be angled 15° to the truncation line in order to ensure that it orientates along 5. The method of determining the truncation orientation is decribed in Section 4.7.

The above describes the manufacturer's recommendations for back surface toric lenses. The end point assumes a non-astigmatic fluid lens and, if only the back surface has been made toric to achieve this, then it follows that this approach allows correction of corneal astigmatism only. The precision and flexibility could perhaps be improved by performing an over-refraction with the fitting set lens in place on the eye, in order to determine more accurately the powers required for the two meridians, and then proceed as above.

5.5.2.2 Front surface torics

The front surface toric contact lens fitting set will consist again of spherical lenses with a truncation and prism. The assessment of the truncation orientation is as described previously in Section 4.7.

(1) Corneal astigmatism

If a fitting set lens is placed on a toric cornea it will warp into a bitoric form and transmit most of the corneal astigmatism. If an over-refraction is performed with this lens, then the optical errors of both principal meridians are revealed. If we regard each meridian as an individual lens then we can see that the problem is no different from that of providing an appropriate soft lens for the spherical cornea of an eye which has no astigmatism. On the flat meridian the soft lens BVP to order is the algebraic addition of the trial contact lens BVP and the effective power of the lens in the refractor head at the cornea. The lens manufacturer simply calculates the front surface radius required for this contact lens, starting out with a back surface power based on the BCOR of the lens. Any power change induced by flexure is already accounted for, since the over-refraction is performed with the lens under the influence of the corneal curves. The above applies equally to the steeper corneal meridian. The over-refraction result here will indicate more myopia and the extra negative power required will result in a front surface for the contact lens which is flatter than that of the less myopic meridian. The lens which is produced for this particular eye will have a spherical back surface and a toric front surface which makes the lens more negative in the most myopic meridian. When this lens is placed on the eye it is assumed that the back surface will warp into a toric form identical with that which was present with the trial lens and so the fluid lens power will be identical with that present at the time of the over-refraction, as will the amount of lens flexure.

An example may clarify the picture. An eye with keratometry readings

8.30 along 5/7.75 along 95

and an ocular refraction of

-6.00 DS/-2.75 DC $\times$ 5

is fitted with a spherical fitting set lens of back optic radius 8.60 mm, BVP -5.50 DS and central thickness 0.3 mm. The over-refraction result is -0.50 DS/-2.50 DC $\times$ 5. What are the front surface radii for this lens assuming the central thickness remains at 0.3 mm?

The over-refraction result in the question is the theoretical result (to the nearest 0.25) assuming a soft lens central thickness of 0.3 mm and a matching fit between the lens back surface and the anterior cornea. If we use Bennett's flexure equation

$$F_V' = -300\, t \left(\frac{1}{r_2'^2} - \frac{1}{r_2^2} \right)$$

(see Section 5.5) then the flexure-induced power change is approximately -0.1 D along 180 and -0.3 D along 90. (The equation was derived assuming a refractive index of 1.44.) Thus we can see that the over-refraction result includes any flexure-induced change in power.

The lens to be ordered would be

back optic radius 8.60, BVP -6.00 DS$/-2.50$ DC $\times 5$

The front surface radii can be calculated using the step along method. In *Figure 5.19*

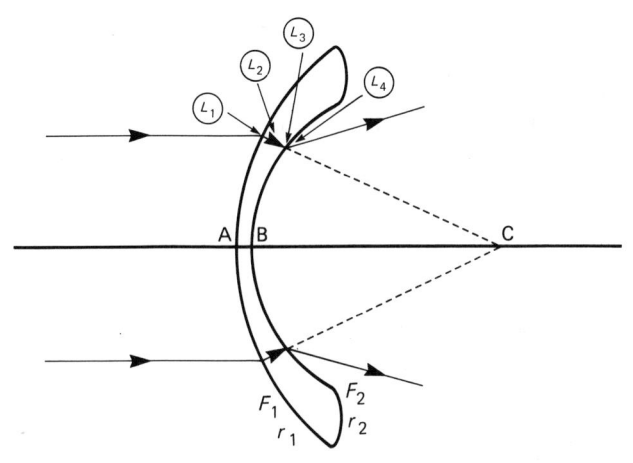

Figure 5.19. Vergence changes in the soft lens.

back surface power $F_2 = \dfrac{1-n}{r_2} = \dfrac{-444}{8.6} = -51.63$ D

reduced thickness $\dfrac{t}{n} = \dfrac{0.3}{1.444} = 0.21$ mm

Along 5

	Vergence (D)	Distance (mm)
BVP = L_4 =	-6.00	
F_2 =	-51.63	
L_3 =	$+45.63$	$\longrightarrow$ 21.92 = BC
		0.21 = t/n
L_2 =	$+45.19$ $\longleftarrow$	22.13 = AC
L_1 =	0.00	

$$\therefore F_1 = +45.19, \; r_1 = \frac{444}{45.19} = 9.83 \text{ mm}$$

Along 95

     Vergence (D) *Distance (mm)*

$\text{BVP} = L_4 = \;\; -8.50$

$F_2 = \underline{-51.63}$

$L_3 = +43.13 \longrightarrow 23.19 = \text{BC}$

          $\underline{0.21} = t/n$

$L_2 = +42.74 \longleftarrow 23.40 = \text{AC}$

$L_1 = \;\; \underline{0.00}$

$$F_1 = +42.74, \; r_1 = \frac{444}{42.74} = 10.39 \text{ mm}$$

(2) Lenticular astigmatism

Since the front surface of the lens is being used to correct the astigmatic error, the lens will correct lenticular astigmatism. If a soft lens rests on an eye which has a spherical cornea but possesses lenticular astigmatism, then it will correct the eye in a very similar way to a front surface toric hard lens. This means that this design can be used for both corneal and lenticular astigmatism or a combination of the two.

5.6 Radial thickness

In the case of hard gas permeable (GPH) and soft lenses an assessment of the oxygen transmission by the lens can only be made if the thickness of the lens is calculated. The edge thickness calculation in Section 2.10 gives axial edge thickness, which is fine from the point of view of checking the specification but is inappropriate for dealing with the problems of gas flow through the material. If we assume that the flow is via the shortest route then we need to calculate radial thickness. This itself must be an approximation since the flow cannot be radial to both surfaces. The standard form of expressing radial thickness is in relation to the lens back surface central radius. This also results in an inappropriate measurement for the periphery of a multicurve or aspheric back surface contact lens since the direction of measurement is not radial to either front or back surface.

The best compromise is probably to measure the lens thickness radially in relation to the front surface of the contact lens. Indeed an international standard on vocabulary and terminology for contact lenses which is currently in preparation will specify that radial edge thickness should be measured normal to the front surface of the lens. The example in Section 2.10 illustrated how to calculate the axial edge thickness and we can use this as a starting point to calculate the radial thickness. *Figure 5.20* illustrates the relationships:

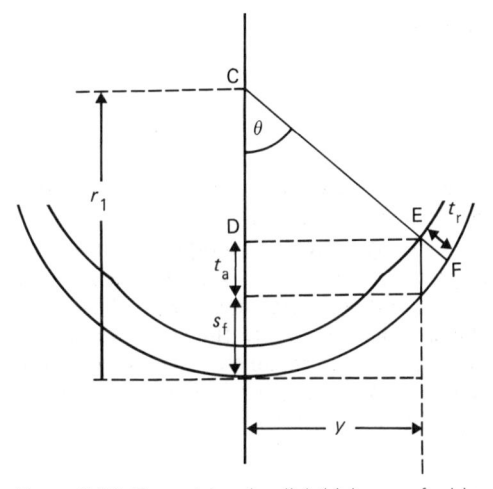

Figure 5.20. The axial and radial thickness of a bicurve contact lens.

$$\tan \theta = \frac{y}{r_1 - t_a - s_f}$$

where r_1 is the radius of curvature of the front surface, t_a is the axial edge thickness and s_f is the sag of the front surface over semi-diameter y. We can therefore deduce the angle θ.

In the triangle CDE

$$\sin \theta = \frac{y}{CE}$$

$$\therefore CE = \frac{y}{\sin \theta}$$

$$t_r = CF - CE$$

and CF is equal to r_1, the radius of curvature of the front surface. If we take the example in Section 2.10 where

$t_a = 0.17$ mm, $y = 4.25$ mm, $r_1 = 8.50$ mm

$s_f = 1.14$ mm

then

$$\tan \theta = \frac{4.25}{8.50 - 0.17 - 1.14} = \frac{4.25}{7.19} = 0.5911$$

$\therefore \theta = 30.59°$

$$CE = \frac{y}{\sin \theta} = \frac{4.25}{0.5089} = 8.3513 \text{ mm}$$

$t_r = 8.5 - 8.3513$

$t_r = 0.149$ mm

In order to use this parameter to assess the oxygen transmission in a lens, it is necessary to make repeated calculations at increasing eccentricities. A computer is ideally suited to this type of problem. There is a computer program in Chapter 7 that performs this function for C2, C3, C4, offset and aspheric back surface lenses.

The practitioner then needs to average the thickness values in order to acquire a mean thickness. The mean thickness is a useful concept as far as the dimensions of the contact lens are concerned; however, Sammons (1981) points out that since gas flow is proportional to $1/t$ we need an average of the $1/t$ values, i.e.

$$\frac{1}{t} \text{ average} = \frac{1/t_1 + 1/t_2 + \ldots 1/t_n}{n}$$

This results in an effective or harmonic mean thickness

$$L = \frac{n}{1/t_1 + 1/t_2 + \ldots 1/t_n}$$

and the harmonic mean thickness is used to assess the gas transmission of a contact lens.

If the oxygen permeability (Dk) of the material is then divided by the harmonic mean thickness (L), we acquire the expression Dk/L which indicates the oxygen transmissibility of the contact lens. Pearson (1986) has reviewed fully the equations employed for both axial and radial thicknesses which include axial/radial conversions and a discussion of the various approaches to the problem of defining average contact lens thickness.

5.7 Summary

- With a front surface solid bifocal it may be necessary to add extra positive power to the addition in order to compensate for the partial neutralization induced by fluid collecting and forming a meniscus on the contact lens front surface.
- With a PMMA back surface solid bifocal the power of the add in air (which will be checked on a focimeter) is 3.18 times the power of the add on the eye.
- The aphakic contact lens wearer may not need a reading addition, owing to the positive spherical abberration of the contact lens which provides extra positive power in the lens periphery.
- In the case of a monocular aphakic the practitioner should bear in mind the possibility of control of the retinal image size by combining the contact lens with a negative spectacle lens.
- For lenticulated lenses for aphakic eyes the junction axial thickness should be around 0.15 mm or larger. The edge thickness should be somewhat larger than this in order to encourage the upper lid to hold the lens in a central position.
- A contact lens/spectacle lens telescope suffers from the restriction of a small lens separation. This results in the lens powers required being high and yet only achieving a modest magnification.
- Flexure of a soft lens results in only a small change of lens power. The power change is independent of the lens BVP but is dependent on lens thickness. Thicker lenses undergo greater power changes and all lenses become more negative with steepening of their surfaces.
- Soft lenses will tend to steepen as their temperature increases and as they dehydrate.
- For toric back surface soft lenses you simply order the smaller surface radius which corrects the ocular corneal astigmatism.
- For toric front surface lenses you simply state the specification of the best fitting trial lens with the over-refraction result which must include the astigmatic component.

6 Checking the lens specification

The topic of lens checking is well covered from a practical point of view in many contact lens textbooks. The reader is particularly recommended to use *Contact Lenses* edited by Stone and Phillips (1980). It is the intention therefore that this chapter will concentrate on the optical principles of the various techniques.

6.1 The optical spherometer

In the UK the optical spherometer is usually called a radiuscope: this name was originally the trade name of the American Optical Company instrument. This instrument may be used to measure both the back and front optic radii and lens thickness. The fundamental working principle is derived from Drysdale's method and is illustrated in *Figure 6.1*.

In *Figure 6.1* the microscope is fitted with a self-luminous target T which is introduced into the main optical system by the semi-silvered mirror M. The microscope objective produces an image of T at T'. If this image is focussed on the surface under examination as in *Figure 6.1(a)*, then the central ray is reflected back along its own path with the left-hand incident ray reflected back along the right-hand ray, and vice versa. These reflected rays will form an image at T. However, since the mirror is semi-silvered, 50% of the light will pass through the mirror to form an image at T″ and this can be observed via the microscope eyepiece. The image T″ is in the first focal plane of the eyepiece which is at the same distance from the mirror centre as the target T. *Figure 6.1(b)* illustrates that an image of the target will also be formed in the first focal plane of the eyepiece when image T' is at the centre of curvature of the surface, since all light rays will strike the surface at normal incidence and will therefore be reflected back up their own paths. The distance between the two positions of the microscope is equal to the radius of curvature of the surface.

If, for example, the concave surface of a contact lens is being examined, the reflections from the convex surface can be eliminated

The optical spherometer 141

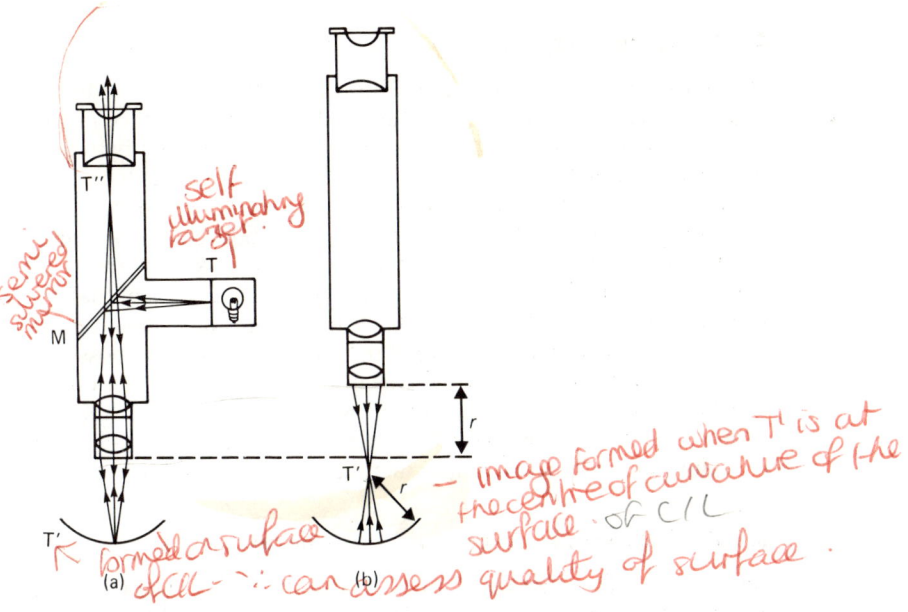

Figure 6.1. The optical spherometer.

by floating the contact lens on a fluid of a refractive index equal to that of the contact lens. From a practical point of view, tap water will reduce the unwanted reflection to an acceptable level. In *Figure 6.1(a)* the image T' is formed on the surface of the lens and, since this surface is seen magnified by courtesy of the microscope, the instrument can be used to assess the quality of the surface. Even superficial scratches, for example, will be obvious. In this position the image T" will not be displaced from the centre of the field of view as the contact lens is horizontally displaced on the microscope table. However, in position (b) the image T' must coincide with the centre of curvature of the contact lens surface. Any horizontal displacement of the lens will result in the image formed by reflection being displaced in the same direction as the lens movement. It is therefore advisable to set the instrument up in position (b) and ensure that the image T" is in the centre of the field of view before attempting a radius measurement.

Figure 6.1 illustrates the instrument being used on a concave surface only; however, it is easy to envisage its use on convex surfaces. The optical spherometer scale divisions are 0.01 mm.

6.1.1 Toric surfaces

In the case of a toric surface, position (*a*) will produce the target image T″ in exactly the same way as a spherical surface since *Figure 6.1(a)* illustrates that the image is theoretically produced by reflection at a point on the surface. Thus the form of the surface (concave; convex; toric; aspheric) is of no significance in this position. However, in position (*b*) the toric surface will produce two principal centres of curvature and the target image T″ will look very similar to a focimeter target seen when examining a sphere/cyl ophthalmic lens. The operator will see line images from point objects and must endeavour to focus the long edge of the line as accurately as possible; this will give the radius value for one of the two principal meridians. Further movement of the microscope will result in the focal lines reforming at 90° to their previous orientation where the radius of curvature of the other principal meridian can be measured.

6.1.2 Aspheric surfaces and peripheral curves

In the case of an aspheric surface we require the vertex radius. Inspection of *Figure 6.1(b)* reveals that a central zone of the contact lens is used to produce the image T″. The diameter of this zone can be reduced by stopping down the aperture of the illuminator. Most instruments are provided with reduced apertures for this purpose and also for measuring the radius of peripheral zones where the width of the surface of interest is small. In this latter case the lens is tilted on the microscope table in order to ensure normal incidence of the light rays in position (*b*).

6.1.3 Thickness measurement

If the contact lens is placed on the microscope table without the use of fluid to minimize reflections from the lower surface, and the microscope is set at position (*a*), then two images will be seen simultaneously. The image formed by the upper surface will be seen clearly and the other slightly blurred image which is formed by reflection from the lower surface can be made clear by a small movement of the microscope in a downward direction. This movement is equal to the apparent central thickness of the contact lens. The real thickness is acquired by multiplying the apparent thickness by the contact lens refractive index. The actual point being investigated can be observed if the instrument is used in a darkened room, since the image T′ is formed on the surface of the lens which acts like a projection screen. Axial edge thickness measurement can be made as above; however, radial edge thickness cannot be measured with any great precision since there is no way of knowing how much lens tilt is required on the microscope table to ensure a truly radial measurement. Pearson (1980) has suggested making an apparent thickness measurement as described above, then making a real thickness measurement by focussing on the contact lens central upper surface and then removing the lens and focussing on the supporting surface. The ratio of the real and apparent thickness provides us with a convenient way of determining the refractive index of the material.

6.1.4 Diameter measurement

Some radiuscopes come equipped with a secondary eyepiece which contains an eyepiece graticule marked off in 0.1 mm divisions. The instrument is then used like a conventional microscope with external illumination. It must be emphasized that the lens image and graticule must coincide; this can be checked by the observer moving the head from side to side, when no parallax between the image and the graticule should be observed.

6.1.5 Edge lift

The optical spherometer can be adapted to measure axial edge lift indirectly. The underlying principle is discussed fully in Section 2.11. Essentially we need to measure only two parameters: the central back surface radius of curvature, and the primary sag of the back surface at a diameter equal to the diameter for the edge lift.

The radial edge lift e can be determined using the equation

$$e = \sqrt{(r-x)^2 + y^2} - r$$

where r is the BCOR and x is the primary sag of the contact lens over a semi-diameter y.

6.1.6 Soft lenses and the wet cell

The flexibility of a soft lens means that the surfaces are likely to warp in air under the influence of gravity. Also the soft lens will be dehydrating during the measurement, which may well alter the surface specification. The lens temperature will be influenced by the air temperature in the checking room and this may not be particularly well controlled. It is thus preferable to check the lens in a wet cell where the fluid supports the lens and maintains full hydration at a steady temperature. The plane surface of the wet cell will refract the emerging light rays and this must be taken into account.

In *Figure 6.2* the optical spherometer target T' (of *Figure 6.1*) will need to be positioned at A' and C'. The microscope movement from position (*a*) to position (*b*) will be the distance A'C'.

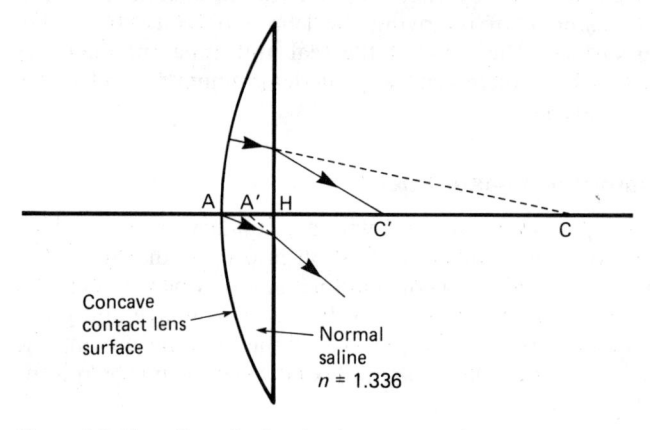

Figure 6.2. The effect of refraction in a wet cell for a light ray directed to the centre of curvature of the surface C and a light ray from the vertex A. AC is the radius of curvature of the concave contact lens surface; A'C' is the apparent radius of curvature measured by the optical spherometer.

The real depth of saline AH is nA'H where n is the refractive index of the saline and A'H is the apparent depth. If we reversed the path of the upper light ray so that we assumed that it was coming from C' in air to be viewed in the normal saline apparently coming from C, then we have the relationship

$$\frac{1}{n} = \frac{\text{real depth}}{\text{apparent depth}} = \frac{\text{HC'}}{\text{HC}}$$

$$\therefore \text{HC} = n\text{HC'}$$

Now from *Figure 6.2*, the radius of curvature of the surface is

$$\text{AC} = \text{AH} + \text{HC}$$

$$\text{AH} + \text{HC} = n\text{A'H} + n\text{HC'} = n(\text{A'H} + \text{HC'})$$

$$= n\text{A'C'}$$

A'C' is the apparent radius of curvature measured by the optical spherometer. Therefore when using an optical spherometer on a soft contact lens in a saline wet cell we must multiply the measured radius by the refractive index of the normal saline, and the precision of the measurement is therefore lowered a little. An optical spherometer has been produced with an objective which can be immersed in a deep saline cell and this avoids the effects of refraction at the plane surface of the wet cell. The movement of this instrument gives a direct reading of the radius of curvature.

The light reflected from the contact lens surface in the wet cell is reduced due to the increasing similarity of the refractive indices of the lens and the normal saline.

Fresnel's law for light of normal incidence is

$$R = \left(\frac{n_L - n_s}{n_L + n_s}\right)^2 \times 100$$

where R is the percentage of reflected light, n_L is the refractive index of the lens and n_s is the refractive index of the saline solution. If n_L is taken to be 1.43 and n_s is 1.336, then R in air is 3.13% and R in the wet cell is 0.115%. Therefore, if an optical spherometer is to be used, the light source will need to have a high light output. Even with this precaution, however, we are faced with two images in close approximation from the two surfaces of the contact lens, and careful considered observation will be needed. Once again the apparent thickness of the lens could be measured with the optical spherometer/wet cell combination.

The soft lens can be measured in air like a hard or GPH lens; however, a suitable holder is needed which allows the lens to be supported by floating it on a saline solution without capillary attraction forces distorting the lens. The surface of interest will require blotting dry and even then the accumulation of surface moisture often precludes a clear image.

6.2 The keratometer

The keratometer can be used to measure concave surfaces; however, since the mire images are formed by reflection at regions of the surface outside the paraxial zone, an allowance must be made during calibration for the non-paraxial nature of the image formation. Bennett (1966) has shown that the difference in the aberrations of convex and concave surfaces can account for the corrections which have to be applied when a keratometer is used to measure the BCOR of a contact lens. Some instrument manufacturers provide conversion tables for concave surfaces. These tables illustrate that the concave surface has a radius of curvature which is longer by 0.02 mm for steep BCORs (6.5 mm), and by up to 0.04 mm for flat BCORs (9.50 mm). Therefore an addition of 0.03 mm to the radius indicated by the keratometer will give a realistic result for the BCOR of the contact lens.

It will be recalled from Section 3.4 that an annulus of approximate diameter 3 mm is used for the generation of the mire images. The keratometer will therefore be unsuitable for measuring intermediate and peripheral radii on a multicurve contact lens and the reading obtained from an aspheric surface will obviously not indicate the vertex radius. On the other hand, a keratometer is likely to give a better indication of the exact orientation of the principal meridians of a toric lens surface. As with the optical spherometer the surface not under investigation is neutralized by floating the lens on a suitable fluid. A 45° mirror or reflecting prism can be used to allow convenient observation of the contact lens by the keratometer. The keratometer radius scale divisions are 0.05 mm.

6.2.1 Scleral lenses

The optic portion of a scleral lens produces no new problems when using a keratometer to check the radius of curvature of the surface. However, the radius of curvature of the scleral portion is likely to be so large as to be off the normal keratometer scale. It will be recalled that in Section 3.7 we observed that a negative auxiliary lens placed in front of the keratometer telescope objective results in the instrument reading steep. This therefore means the keratometer can now be used for measuring flat radii. Usually a -1.00 D or -2.00 D trial case lens will be used, with the practitioner deriving a conversion table from measurements made on steel balls of accurately known diameter. It goes without saying that a positive auxiliary lens of similar power can be used for steep radii, most commonly encountered in keratoconic cases and when measuring soft lenses in a wet cell.

6.2.2 Soft lenses

If the soft lens is suitably prepared and suitably supported, then a keratometer like the optical spherometer can be used to measure the BCOR of the soft lens in air. However, as with the spherometer, the result is more likely to be truly representative if the lens remains fully supported, fully hydrated and at a controlled temperature in a saline

The keratometer 147

wet cell, where the radius indicated by the instrument will require multiplying by the refractive index of the saline solution.

If, for the sake of simplicity, we assume that the keratometer is a telecentric instrument, then in *Figure 6.3(a)* the mire image h_1'

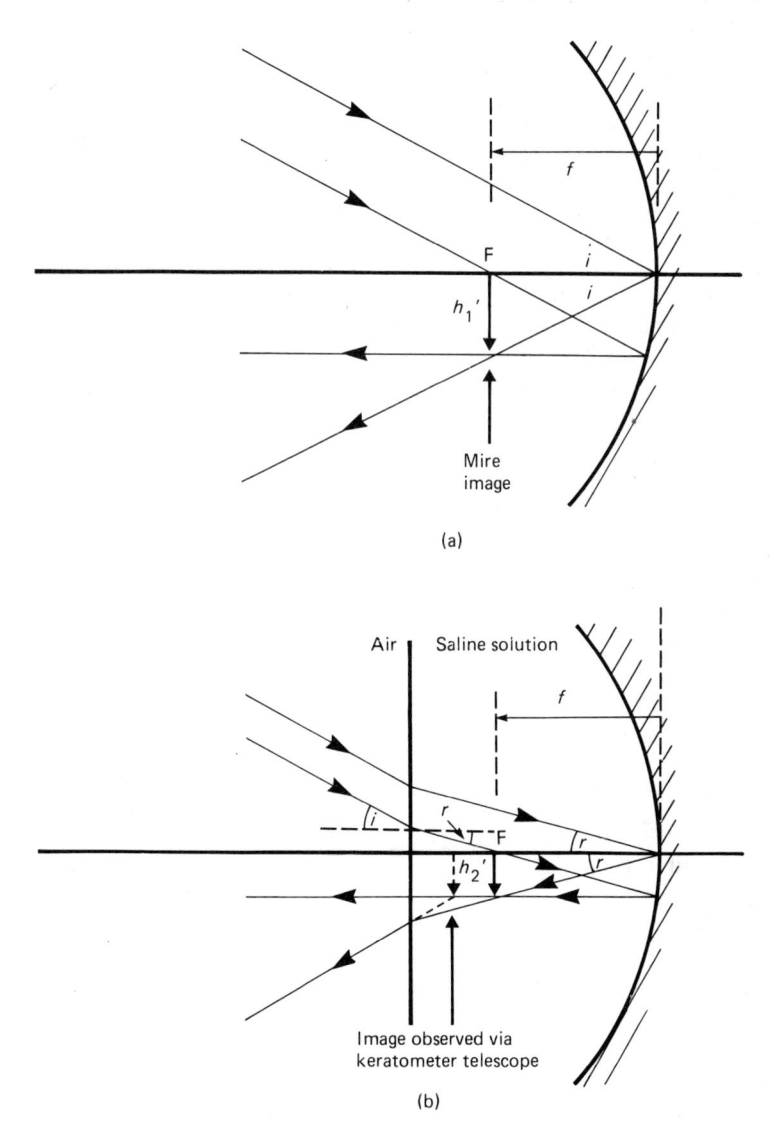

(a)

(b)

Figure 6.3. Keratometer image formation (a) in air and (b) in a wet cell.

produced by reflection in the contact lens surface will be in the focal plane F. Since

$$\tan i = \frac{h_1'}{f}$$

the image size is

$$h_1' = f \tan i \tag{6.1}$$

If the same lens is placed in a wet cell, as in *Figure 6.3(b)*, then the angle of incidence i is reduced by refraction at the air/saline boundary to the angle of refraction r. The pencil of light rays within the saline solution is still parallel and so the point image will form as before in the focal plane F; however, the reduction of angle i to angle r ensures that the image size h_2' is smaller than that formed when the lens was in air. *Figure 6.3(b)* also shows that the size h_2' is the size of the image which is observed via the keratometer telescope. The keratometer must be moved away from the lens a little to maintain a correct focus at the eyepiece. Since

$$\tan r = \frac{h_2'}{f}$$

the image size in the wet cell is

$$h_2' = f \tan r \tag{6.2}$$

Therefore, from (6.1) and (6.2)

$$\frac{h_1'}{\tan i} = \frac{h_2'}{\tan r}$$

$$\therefore h_2' = \frac{\tan r}{\tan i} h_1'$$

For small angles

$$\frac{\tan r}{\tan i} = \frac{\sin r}{\sin i} = \frac{1}{n}$$

where n is the refractive index of the saline solution. So the image size in the wet cell is

$$h_2' = \frac{h_1'}{n}$$

The keratometer equation derived in Section 3.2 is

radius of curvature $= -2\dfrac{h_1'}{h_1}d$

The wet cell reduces h_1' to h_1'/n. It therefore follows that the radius of curvature indicated by the instrument will be reduced to (radius)/n. Thus the radius of curvature given by the instrument when a wet cell is employed must be multiplied by the refractive index of the saline solution. All the above has neglected to include the correction factor of $+0.03$ mm required for concave surfaces. Since the wet cell results in steep radius measurements it may be more appropriate to add 0.02 mm to the indicated radius, so that if the keratometer reads 6.22 mm we must apply the correction factor of $+0.02$ mm, giving 6.24 mm, and this must be multiplied by the refractive index of the saline solution.

$$\therefore \text{BCOR} = 6.24 \times 1.336 = 8.34 \text{ mm}$$

As with the optical spherometer the surface reflections are severely reduced and so the mire luminosity must be increased considerably, and even then the practitioner must cope with an image formed by each of the two contact lens surfaces. The image formed by the surface which is nearest to the mires will be the brightest and the smaller of the two images will be produced by the steeper of the two surfaces.

6.3 The spherometer

The problems described above make the use of the optical spherometer or keratometer a less than attractive proposition. One of the most popular approaches to the problem of measuring the BCOR of a soft contact lens is to use a spherometer. This is simply an instrument that measures the sag of a given chord and from this the radius of curvature of the surface can be deduced. This is the fundamental working principle of the lens measure.

In the contact lens field the instrument, which can be wet or dry cell, is as illustrated in *Figure 6.4*. The moving micrometer probe is raised until it just touches the back surface of the contact lens and this gives the sag which is converted to radius of curvature as shown below. In *Figure 6.5*, from Pythagoras' theorem,

$r^2 = y^2 + (r-s)^2$

$\therefore r^2 = y^2 + r^2 - 2rs + s^2$

$\therefore 0 = y^2 - 2rs + s^2$

150 Checking the lens specification

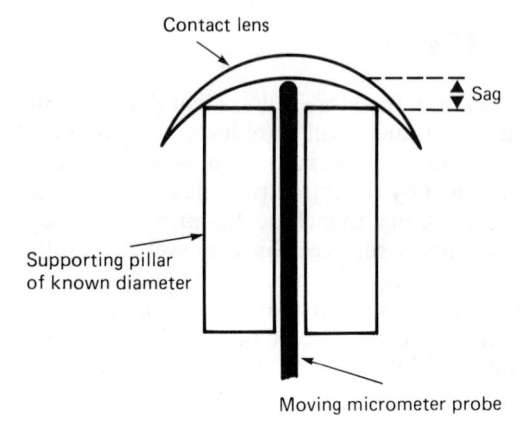

Figure 6.4. The spherometer. The moving probe measures the sag of the surface over the pillar diameter.

$$\therefore 2rs = y^2 + s^2$$

$$r = \frac{y^2 + s^2}{2s}$$

The point of contact between the spherometer probe and the lens surface can be observed by viewing a magnified sagittal section of the lens as it sits on the supporting pillar. When contact has been made, any further raising of the probe will induce movement of the contact lens. The micrometer adjustment screw gives a BCOR to a claimed accuracy of ±0.1 mm. This system allows measurement of lens thickness and diameter.

As already stated, this approach can be used with a wet cell or dry cell technique. The problems associated with dry cells have already been listed; however, as far as spherometry is concerned there is another which is associated with the lack of physical support for the lens. This results in a positive-powered lens with its greatest thick-

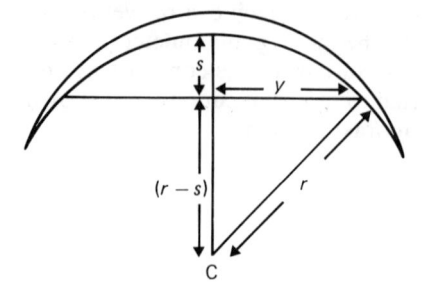

Figure 6.5. The principle of the spherometer. C is the centre of curvature of the back surface of the contact lens of radius r and sag s over a semi-diamater y.

ness at the lens centre tending to warp into a flatter form. The negative lens, on the other hand, with its thick edge hanging off the sides of the supporting pillar will tend to warp into a steeper form. For all lenses, whether wet or dry cell, it is important to centralize the lens on the supporting pillar. Some instruments incorporate devices to help with this centration. As an alternative to observing the point of contact between the probe and the lens surface, some instruments utilize the electrical conductivity of the soft lens with the point of contact completing an electrical circuit, which results in the activation of a light emitting diode or the digital display of the surface radius. Alternatively an ultrasonic system can be used to measure the sag.

6.4 The focimeter

The focimeter provides the optometrist with an accurate and convenient method of determining the back vertex power (BVP) of any ophthalmic lens. The lens under examination must rest against the focimeter stop. If the back surface of the lens is in contact with the stop then the end point will give the BVP. The assumption is made that the back vertex of the lens coincides with the plane of the stop. A typical contact lens possesses surfaces which are very steeply curved and so the above assumption may introduce significant errors when a standard focimeter stop is used as in *Figure 6.6(a)*,

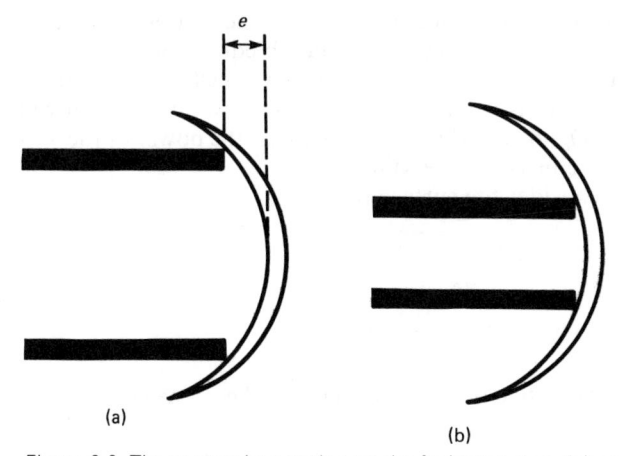

Figure 6.6. The contact lens resting on the focimeter stop: (a) standard focimeter stop diameter; (b) reduced focimeter stop diameter for contact lens work.

which illustrates that the contact lens back vertex is e mm to the right of the focimeter stop. In this case the focimeter reading at the end point will be the effective power of the lens e mm from the back surface. For a positive contact lens the focimeter will give a power which is greater than the BVP, with the power being less than the BVP for a negative lens. The discrepancy will become more and more significant as the contact lens power is increased. The problem is minimized as shown in *Figure 6.6(b)* by fitting a reduced diameter stop to the focimeter. Many focimeters are provided with a reduced diameter stop as a standard accessory. If the lens is turned around so that the lens front surface rests against the stop, then the focimeter will indicate the front vertex power (FVP), but the standard diameter stop will result in the lens front vertex being to the left of the plane of the stop. This means that for a positive lens the focimeter reading will be less than the lens FVP. Once again this effect is minimized with the small diameter stop.

6.4.1 Soft lenses

The soft lens BVP can be measured in air provided certain precautions are taken. A projection focimeter should be used if possible with the power scale set at the expected reading. The lens surfaces should be carefully dried and the reading taken as soon as possible, although Mandell (1974) has suggested that shrinkage on dehydration does not substantially affect the readings for about 4 min. A reliability around ±0.25 D is claimed; however, the lens is subjected to the environmental influences described in the sections on radius measurement (Sections 6.1 and 6.2). Undoubtedly a soft lens will be in a more stable state if examined in a wet cell. Once again a projection focimeter is recommended. The lens/wet cell system will be as shown in *Figure 6.7* which illustrates that the power of the lens is dramatically reduced by the saline cell.

Let us now consider the surface powers.

Front surface
In air

$$F_1 = \frac{n-1}{r_1}$$

where n is the refractive index of the lens. In the saline cell

$$F_1 = \frac{n-n_s}{r_1}$$

where n_s is the refractive index of the saline solution. Therefore

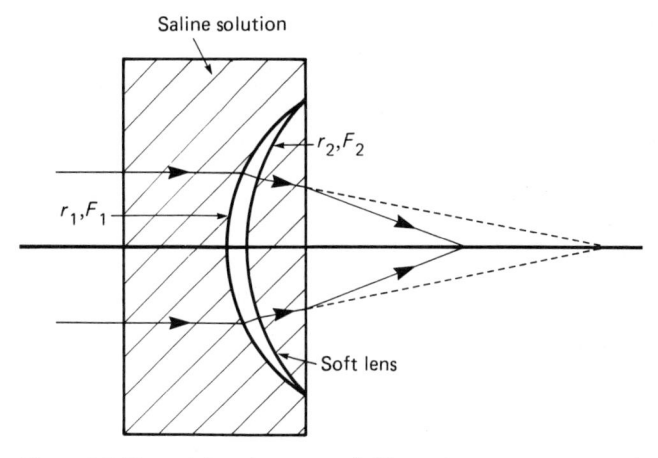

Figure 6.7. The soft lens in a wet cell. The surface powers are much reduced due to being in contact with the saline solution.

$$\frac{F_1(\text{air})}{F_1(\text{saline})} = \frac{n-1}{r_1}\frac{r_1}{n-n_s} = \frac{n-1}{n-n_s}$$

$$\therefore F_1(\text{air}) = \frac{n-1}{n-n_s}F_1(\text{saline})$$

If we take n as 1.444 and n_s as 1.336, then

surface power in air = surface power in saline × 4.111

We can therefore state that the power in the saline cell will be approximately one-quarter of the power in air.

Back surface
The above relationship will hold for the back surface power F_2, and if we consider the contact lens to be a thin lens then

BVP = $F_1 + F_2$

∴ BVP in air = BVP in saline × 4.111

However, this does not hold for a thick lens system.
Suppose the soft lens has a BCOR of 8.30 mm, a central thickness t_c of 0.3 mm, a front surface radius r_1 of 7.10 mm and a refractive index n of 1.444.

BVP in air
In *Figure 6.8*

$$F_1 = \frac{444}{7.1} = +62.54 \text{ D}$$

$$F_2 = \frac{-444}{8.3} = -53.49 \text{ D}$$

$t/n = 0.21$ mm

	Vergence (D)		Distance (mm)	
$L_1 =$	0.00			
$F_1 =$	$+62.54$			
$L_2 =$	$+62.54 \longrightarrow \frac{1000}{62.54} \longrightarrow$		15.99	= AC
			-0.21	$= t/n$
$L_3 =$	$+63.37 \longleftarrow \frac{1000}{15.78} \longleftarrow$		15.78	= BC
$F_2 =$	-53.49			
$L_4 =$	$+9.88 =$ BVP in air			

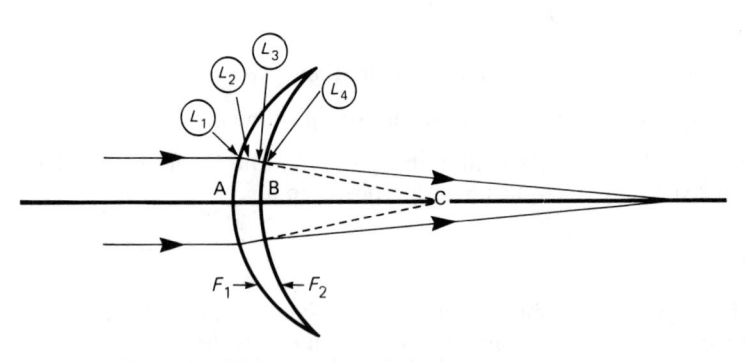

Figure 6.8. The path of light rays through the lens.

BVP in saline solution
In *Figure 6.8*

$$F_1 = \frac{108}{7.1} = +15.21 \text{ D}$$

$$F_2 = \frac{-108}{8.3} = -13.01 \text{ D}$$

$t/n = 0.21$ mm

	Vergence (D)		Distance (mm)
$L_1 =$	0.00		
$F_1 =$	$+15.21$		
$L_2 =$	$+15.21 \longrightarrow \frac{1000}{15.21} \longrightarrow$		$65.75 =$ AC
			$-0.21 = t/n$
$L_3 =$	$+15.26 \longleftarrow \frac{1000}{65.54} \longleftarrow$		$65.54 =$ BC
$F_2 =$	-13.01		
$L_4 =$	$+2.25 =$ BVP in saline		

If

BVP in air = BVP in saline × 4.11

BVP in air = $+2.25 \times 4.11$

$\qquad = +9.25$ D

Clearly this produces an unacceptable error since the BVP in air was found to be $+9.88$ D.

If we return to *Figure 6.7* we can see that one further problem remains and that is that light will be refracted at the plane saline/air boundary. Let us continue with the example above. We have calculated that the BVP in saline is $+2.25$ D. The light will travel from the back vertex of the lens to the saline/air boundary, a distance equal to the sag of the lens.

Let us assume for the sake of simplicity that the lens has a monocurve back surface of BCOR 8.3 mm and diameter 13 mm; then

$$\text{sag} = r - \sqrt{r^2 - y^y}$$
$$= 8.3 - \sqrt{8.3^2 - 6.5^2}$$

sag = 3.14 mm

reduced sag $\dfrac{s}{n} = \dfrac{3.14}{1.336} = 2.35$ mm

156 Checking the lens specification

$$\text{BVP} = +2.25 \xrightarrow[\text{Vergence (D)}]{\dfrac{1000}{2.25}} 444.44 \text{ \textit{Distance (mm)}}$$

$$-2.35 = \text{reduced sag}$$

$$+2.26 \xleftarrow{\dfrac{1000}{442.09}} 442.09$$

Therefore the vergence of light emerging from the posterior plane saline/air boundary is +2.26 D.

We can see that in fact there are two factors to consider. Not only is there some refraction at the saline/air boundary but, assuming that this boundary rests against the focimeter stop, the back vertex of the lens is distanced from the focimeter stop plane. However, since the saline cell has partially neutralized the lens surface powers, this results in the system power being low and consequently these factors do not contribute any significant error. By far the greatest disadvantage of this approach is that the focimeter is working at reduced accuracy. In our example above, the lens in air required a 9.88 D movement of the power scale, but in the saline cell the same lens requires a movement of only 2.25 D, which indicates that the focimeter scale divisions of 0.25 D represent 1.00 D approximately when the wet cell is used. With this in mind the original approximation that the BVP in air equals the BVP in saline multiplied by four can be used practically; however, the resulting measurement is likely to lack precision.

The partial neutralization of the surface powers by the saline will be accompanied by a similar partial neutralization of surface irregularities or unwanted cylinders or prisms.

6.4.2 The radius checking device

The focimeter can be adapted to measure the radius of curvature of the concave surfaces of PMMA corneal contact lenses by incorporation of the radius checking (RC) device developed by Sarver and Kerr (1964). The device is made from PMMA with a refractive index of 1.490 and is as illustrated in *Figure 6.9*. The convex surface has a radius r of 8.87 mm which gives it a power of

$$\frac{490}{8.87} = +55.24 \text{ D}$$

This surface is allowed to rest against the focimeter stop. The

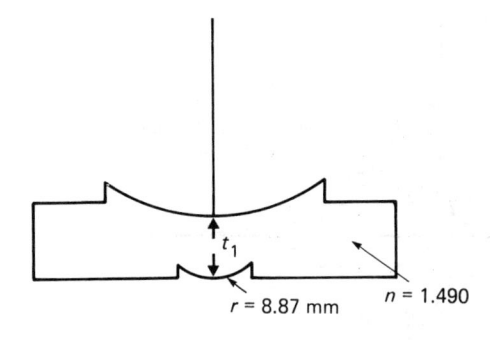

Figure 6.9. The RC device in cross section.

r = 8.87 mm   n = 1.490

focimeter optical axis must be vertical. The contact lens under examination is placed concave surface upward onto the upper concave dish of the device floating on a *small* quantity of fluid of refractive index 1.490. If the RC device has a thickness t_1 and the contact lens has a central thickness t_2 with a BCOR of r_2 then we have in the focimeter a thick lens with surface radii r and r_2 and central thickness $t_1 + t_2$. The focimeter measures the FVP (if we consider that the convex surface is the front surface). We know the power of one surface and the lens central thickness; it is therefore an easy matter to deduce the power and the radius of the other surface. Let us take an example.

Suppose the RC device thickness t_1 is 1.5 mm and the lens under examination has a central thickness of 0.2 mm with a BCOR (r_2) which is unknown. If the focimeter reads +2.75 D, what is the BCOR of the contact lens?

In *Figure 6.10* the focimeter reads +2.75 D.

∴ Vergence $L_1 = -2.75$ D

$t = t_1 + t_2$, $t/n = 1.14$ mm

	Vergence (D)		Distance (mm)	
$L_1 =$	−2.75			
$F_1 =$	+55.24			
$L_2 =$	+52.49	— $\dfrac{1000}{52.49}$ →	19.05	= AC
			−1.14	= t/n
$L_3 =$	+55.83 ←	$\dfrac{1000}{17.91}$ —	17.91	= BC
$L_4 =$	00.00			
$F_2 =$	−55.83			

158 Checking the lens specification

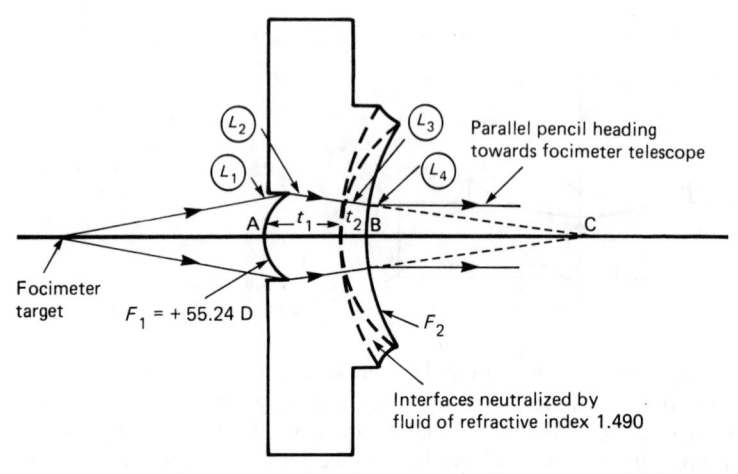

Figure 6.10. The RC device and its effect on the incident pencil of light rays from the focimeter target.

Power of the back surface of the contact lens = -55.83 D

$$\therefore \text{BCOR} = \frac{1-n}{F_2} = \frac{-490}{-55.83} = 8.78 \text{ mm}$$

The calculation can be made more convenient by using the equation which reflects the relationship between front and back surfaces derived in Section 2.3.

It will be recalled that we start off by assuming that the above system is thin and we calculate the BCOR for a thin lens. We then apply the correction factor $\{(n-1)/n\}t$ where t is the central thickness of the system, and since we are concerned with the radius of the back surface we subtract the correction factor from the thin lens radius. In *Figure 6.10*

$L_1 = -2.75$ D

$F_1 = +55.24$ D

$L_2 = +52.49$ D $= L_3$ for a thin lens

$L_4 = 0.00$

$\therefore F_2 = -52.49$ D

$$r_2 = \frac{1-n}{F_2} = \frac{-490}{-52.49} = 9.34 \text{ mm}$$

For a thick lens

$$\text{BCOR} = r_2 - \frac{n-1}{n}t$$

$$= 9.34 - 0.33t$$

$$= 9.34 - 0.56$$

$$= 8.78 \text{ mm}$$

If the above exercise is repeated for a focimeter reading of +3.00 D then the BCOR works out to be 8.82 mm, i.e. a radius change of 0.04 mm. This gives some idea of the sensitivity of the instrument since the focimeter is usually calibrated in 0.25 D steps. There is a computer program in Chapter 7 which calculates the BCOR from the focimeter reading.

6.5 The pachometer

This instrument has already been described in Section 3.13, where its major application was seen to be in measuring corneal thickness and monitoring corneal thickness changes. It could also be used to measure contact lens thickness. The pachometer holds promise as a means of measuring axial edge thickness or axial edge clearance on the eye. It is possible to specify with this instrument (suitably adapted) the exact location of the thickness measurement. This is not possible with any precision using a dial gauge, which measures the edge thickness in a more or less radial direction. The question is, however, 'Radial to what?' Is the edge thickness radial to the back surface or the front surface, or is it somewhere between the two? It most certainly is not radial to the back central optic curve and the dial gauge is therefore of limited value to the practitioner for measuring edge thickness.

Guillon *et al.* (1986) have modified a slit lamp to register the exact location of the pachometer measurement from the lens edge. It is therefore possible to specify with some precision the axial edge thickness and its location. If this approach were used at, say, three or four agreed distances from the edge of the lens then we would have a means of specifying and checking the form of the lens edge.

6.6 The primary optic diameter of a scleral lens

The primary optic diameter (POD) may be stated when ordering a scleral contact lens. The dimension is illustrated in *Figure 6.11* where it can be seen that the POD is the diameter of the transition between the optic and scleral portions of the lens. This, however, is not usually available for direct inspection on a finished lens because of a transition curve being worked on the lens between the optic and scleral curves.

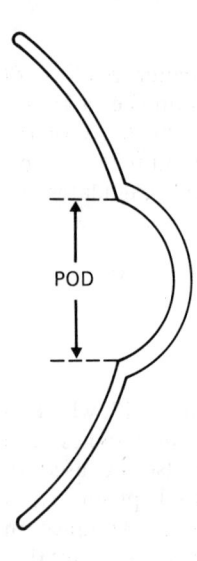

Figure 6.11. The primary optic diameter of a scleral lens.

It can be measured indirectly as follows. In *Figure 6.12*, $2y$ is the primary optic diameter. We can measure A and $2r_s$, where r_s is the radius of curvature of the scleral back surface. We can measure t_c, and we can deduce s from

$$s = A - 2r_s - t_c$$

but

$$s = s_2 - s_1 = \left(r_0 - \sqrt{r_0^2 - y^2}\right) - \left(r_s - \sqrt{r_s^2 - y^2}\right)$$

where r_0 is the radius of curvature of the back surface of the optic. The only unknown quantity in this equation is y.

Let us take an example. Suppose s is found to be 1.3 mm for a lens

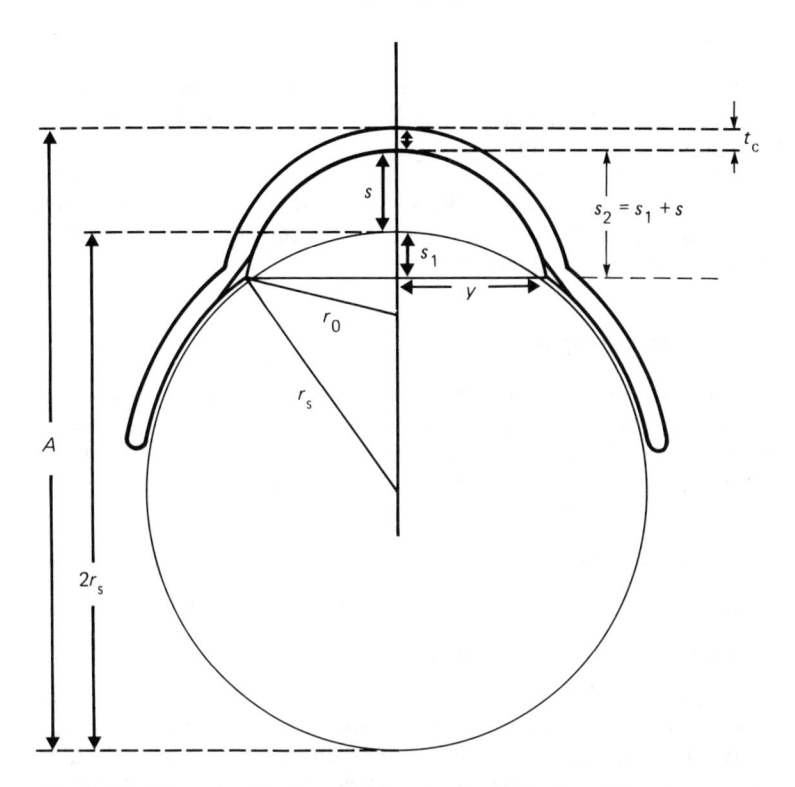

Figure 6.12. The scleral lens mounted on a sphere of radius of curvature equal to that of the scleral curve.

with a back optic radius r_0 of 8.0 mm and a scleral radius of 13.0 mm. Substituting in the equation above we have

$$s = 8 - \sqrt{8^2 - y^2} - 13 + \sqrt{13^2 - y^2}$$

$$s = 8 - \sqrt{64 - y^2} - 13 + \sqrt{169 - y^2}$$

At this stage the easiest approach is to use an iterative treatment where we substitute the expected POD into the equation. If we assume that the POD is 12 mm then

$y = 6$ mm

and s works out at 1.24 mm which is less than the 1.3 mm acquired by measurement. If we assume that the POD is 12.2 mm then

$y = 6.1$ mm

and s works out at 1.3 mm which is equal to that found by measurement. We thus deduce that the POD of this lens by indirect measurement is 12.2 mm.

From the above we can see that in this example a 0.1 mm change in POD will be accompanied by an approximate change of 0.03 mm in the value of s. This gives us some idea of the precision required in making the measurements A, $2r_s$ and t_c.

6.7 Tolerances

At the time of writing, the British Standard dealing with tolerances is being rewritten. However, it may appear somewhat parochial to consider only the British recommendations for allowable tolerances when checking the specification of a contact lens. The writer has therefore consulted:

American National Standard Z80.2—1972 (ANS)

Standards Association of Australia AS 1887—1976 (AS)

British Standards Association BS 5562—1978 (BS)

A comparison of the above bodies may provide the reader with more insight into the validity of the recommendations made by each individual association. The object of specifying tolerances should be to ensure that the product is sufficiently accurate to fulfil its function. There is no point in working to greater accuracy, even if it is technically possible, since this inevitably increases costs to no advantage. A tolerance of ±0.05 mm on the diameter of a hydrated soft lens, for example, is very difficult (if not impossible) to achieve and many practitioners would no doubt feel that the diameter of a hydrated soft lens does not require that degree of precision in order to ensure an acceptable performance and reproducibility on reordering.

The lens parameters to which tolerances have been recommended follow below. The common tolerances are summarized in *Tables 6.1, 6.2* and *6.3*. BS recommends that lenses be tested at a room temperature of 20 ± 0.5°C.

6.7.1 Corneal lenses

BCOR
There is general agreement for this particular parameter, AS and BS suggesting ±0.02 mm, and ANS suggesting ±0.025 mm.

Tolerances 163

Table 6.1 Comparison of tolerances specified for hard corneal lenses

Dimension	Dimensional tolerances (mm)		
	BS 5562 1978	ANS Z80.2 1972	AS 1887 1976
Back central optic radius	±0.02	±0.025	±0.02
Back central optic radius for toroidal surfaces:			
$0 < \Delta r < 0.2$	Not specified	±0.02	±0.02
$0.2 < \Delta r < 0.4$		±0.03	±0.03
$0.4 < \Delta r < 0.6$		±0.05	±0.05
$\Delta r > 0.6$		±0.07	±0.07
Back central optic diameter	±0.20	Light blend: ±0.10 Heavy blend: ±0.20	Light blend: ±0.05 Heavy blend: ±0.10
Peripheral optic radius	±0.10	±0.10	±0.10
Back peripheral diameter	±0.20	Light blend: ±0.05 Heavy blend: ±0.10	±0.05
Total diameter	±0.10	±0.05	±0.05
Front central optic diameter	±0.20	±0.10	±0.10
Bifocal segment height	±0.10	−0.1 to +0.2	−0.1 to +0.2
Centre thickness	±0.02	Less than ±0.02	±0.02
Edge thickness	±0.02		±0.02

Optical property specified	Optical tolerances (D, Δ or degrees)		
Back vertex power:			
+10 to −10	±0.12	±0.12	±0.12
over 10	±0.25	±0.25	±0.25
Cylinder power:			
less than 2.00	±0.25	±0.25	±0.25
2.00 to 4.00	±0.37	±0.37	±0.37
over 4.00	±0.50	±0.50	±0.50
Cylinder axis	±5	±5	Cyl power <1: ±5 Cyl power >1: ±2.5
Prism measured at geometric centre of optic zone	±0.50	Lens power +10 to −10: ±0.25 more than ±10: ±0.50	±0.25
Back vertex power of bifocal addition	Not directly specified	±0.25	±0.25

Table 6.2 Comparison of tolerances specified for hard scleral lenses

Dimension	Dimensional tolerances (mm)		
	BS 5562 1978	ANS Z80.2 1972	AS 1887 1976
Back central optic radius	±0.05	±0.03	±0.03
Back central optic diameter	±0.20	Not specified	±0.10
Back scleral radius (of preformed lens)	±0.10	Not specified	±0.10
Basic or primary optic diameter	±0.10	Not specified	
Peripheral optic radius	±0.10	Not specified	
Back peripheral optic diameter	±0.20 (for preformed lenses)	Not specified	
Total diameter	±0.25	±0.50	±0.50
Back central optic diameter	±0.20	Not specified	
Centre thickness	±0.03	±0.03	±0.03
Vertex clearance from cast	±0.02	±0.02	±0.02

Optical property specified	Optical tolerances (D, Δ or degrees)		
Back vertex power (in the weaker meridian)	+10.0 to −10: ±0.12 Over ±10: ±0.25	±0.12 ±0.25	±0.12 ±0.25
Cylinder power:			
less than 2.00	±0.25		
2.00 to 4.00	±0.37	Not specified	
over 4.00	±0.50		
Cylinder axis	±5	±5	±5
Prism at geometrical centre of optic zone	±0.50	±0.25	±0.25
Optical centration	±0.5 mm	Not specified	

The recommended method of measurement is to use an optical spherometer calibrated to read to 0.01 mm. Alternatively a keratometer could be used (with a suitable conversion scale for concave surfaces); however, most keratometers have a radius scale which is calibrated in 0.05 mm divisions, and may lack the precision required. Other methods of measurement have been suggested, e.g. interfero-

Table 6.3 Comparison of tolerances specified for soft lenses

Dimension	Dimensional tolerances (mm)	
	BS 5562 1978	AS 1887 1976
Back central optic radius	±0.10 (dry) ±0.20 (hydrated)	±0.05 mm (hydrated)
Back central optic diameter	±0.10 (dry)	Not specified
Peripheral optic radius	±0.10 (dry) ±0.20 (hydrated)	Not specified
Back peripheral optic diameter	±0.20 (dry)	Not specified
Total diameter	±0.25 (hydrated)	<50% water content: ±0.05 (hydrated) ⩾50% water content: ±0.10 (hydrated)
Front central optic diameter	±0.20 (dry or hydrated)	Not specified
Centre thickness	±0.02 (dry) ±0.05 (hydrated)	±0.02 (hydrated)
Edge thickness	±0.02 (dry) ±0.05 (hydrated)	Not specified

Optical property specified	Optical tolerances (D, Δ or degrees)	
Back vertex power (in the weaker meridian)	0 to 10: ±0.25 Over 10: ±0.50 (hydrated)	0 to 10: ±0.12 Over 10: ±0.25 (hydrated)
Prism at geometrical centre of optic zone	±0.50 (hydration not specified)	±0.25 (hydrated)
Cylinder power	±0.50 ±0.75 } hydrated ±1.00	Not specified
Cylinder axis	±5	±5

American National Standard Z80.2—1972 does not specify tolerances for soft lenses.

metry, but these are unlikely to be used in clinical practice. The Americans make the point that the accuracy of any measuring system must exceed the prescribed tolerance by a substantial margin.

The ANS recommend that surface uniformity is checked at various points from lens centre to lens edge with curvature variations not exceeding ±0.025 mm radius for the back surface; ±0.02 mm radius for the front surface of a negative lens; and ±0.01 mm radius for the front surface of a positive lens.

BPORs
The universally recommended tolerance is ±0.1 mm. The Americans consider that there is currently no suitable clinical instrumentation for measuring this parameter; however, instruments which operate on the moiré fringe phenomenon could be used for this measurement. The Australians suggest the peripheral radii are measured prior to blending. An optical spherometer can be used to measure peripheral radii, where the peripheral curve has a reasonably large bandwidth. It is necessary to use a small aperture so that light falls onto the contact lens surface within the bandwidth of the curve.

BCOD
ANS stipulate a tolerance which is dependent on the amount of blending at the transition:

±0.1 mm for light blending

±0.2 mm for heavy blending

AS sensibly adopt the same scheme but their tolerances are tighter at

±0.05 mm for light blending

±0.1 mm for heavy blending

BS recommend

±0.2 mm

The recommended method of measurement is to use a 10× magnifying lens in combination with a graticule, or a projection magnification system.

BPODs
Once again ANS fix their tolerances according to the amount of blending at the transition. ANS stipulate

±0.05 mm for light blending

±0.1 mm for heavy blending

AS stipulate

±0.05 mm

BS stipulate

±0.2 mm

The recommended method of measurement is as for the BCOD, a 10× magnifying lens with a graticule, or a projection magnifying system.

OS

The overall size tolerance recommended by all but BS is

±0.05 mm

BS stipulate

±0.1 mm

Once again the method of measurement recommended is by observation with a measuring magnifier. This particular diameter can also be measured with a V gauge and this method is also recommended.

BVP

ANS, AS and BS recommend the following tolerances:

| for BVP up to 10 D | ±0.12 D |
| for BVP greater than 10 D | ±0.25 D |

ANS stipulate that if the BCOR and BVP errors are cumulative then the cumulative error shall not exceed 0.25 D. The cumulative errors in power between the right and left lenses shall not exceed 0.25 D.

AS recommend that the arithmetic difference between the BVP error of the right and left lenses should not exceed 0.25 D or the tolerance specified.

The recommended method of measurement is, of course, by focimeter. ANS recommend a 6 mm aperture with the lens not hand held. AS and BS recommend a focimeter aperture of not less than 4 mm. ANS suggest that a standard technique should be developed for measuring the modulation transfer function and standards established for contact lenses.

AS lay down a specification for the material used for corneal lenses. Clear sheets of the material 0.1 mm thick should have a luminous transmittance of not less than 88% using CIE illuminant 1C, and the refractive index variation should not be greater than 0.5% of the nominated value.

Prism

ANS recommend the following prism tolerances:

for BVP up to 10 D ±0.25 Δ
for BVP greater than 10 D ±0.50 Δ

AS recommend

±0.25 Δ

BS recommend

±0.50 Δ

The method of measurement is by focimeter with the recommendations that are given for BVP measurement. The prism is to be measured at the geometric centre of the optic zone.

Cylinder power
There is universal agreement on the tolerance of cylinder power, as follows:

for cylinder power below 2 D ±0.25 D
for cylinder power of 2–4 D ±0.37 D
for cylinder power over 4 D ±0.50 D

with a tolerance on the cylinder axis of ±5°.

The only exception here are AS who stipulate a tolerance on the axis of ±2.5° where the cylinder power is over 1 D.

The method of measurement is by focimeter as above, with the cyl axis measured relative to a prism base apex line where a ballasting prism is present (this is assumed to be vertical) or relative to the flat meridian of the toric back surface.

Toric surface radii
There is a general agreement on tolerances for this parameter, from ANS and AS:

for radius difference less than
0.2 mm ±0.02 mm
for radius difference of 0.2–
0.4 mm ±0.03 mm
for radius difference of 0.4–
0.6 mm ±0.05 mm
for radius difference greater
than 0.6 mm ±0.07 mm

Central thickness
All three organizations agree and recommend a tolerance of ±0.02 mm. AS also add that the arithmetic difference in thickness error between right and left lenses shall not exceed 0.02 mm.

The recommended method of measurement is to use a measuring dial gauge which is calibrated to 0.01 mm and reads accurately to 0.005 mm.

Edge thickness

This parameter presents more problems than the centre thickness measurement. We must first define whether we wish to measure axial edge thickness or radial edge thickness. The dial gauge is more likely to give a radial thickness measurement but the question arises, 'Radial to what curve?' It is undoubtedly less confusing to use the concept of axial edge thickness and this may in the end be the easiest measurement to make.

Only AS and BS give a recommended tolerance of ±0.02 mm and suggest that the measurement is made with a dial gauge, which makes the measurement difficult to define since it is not precisely radial to the central curve and it most certainly is not an axial measurement. BS also suggest the possibility of using an optical spherometer for edge thickness measurement. This could result in an axial edge thickness value.

Edge form

This most important feature of the lens lacks a suitably precise tolerance. At the moment the edge form is simply described 'as specified' and this is totally inadequate. The Americans and Australians have suggested measuring the edge thickness at three or four distances from the lens edge, and the Australians in particular are developing precise techniques for this approach. This work should be welcomed by the contact lens practitioner.

FCOR

ANS recommend the tolerance is

for negative power lenses	±0.02 mm
for positive power lenses	±0.01 mm

AS recommend a tolerance of

±0.01 mm

This should be measured using an optical spherometer.

It could be argued that this parameter does not need checking directly since it is checked indirectly by checking BCOR, centre thickness, and BVP. Indeed the optometrist is unlikely to specify the FCOR but will probably specify the three parameters above.

FCOD

Where this is present, ANS and AS stipulate a tolerance of

±0.1 mm

BS stipulate a tolerance of

±0.2 mm

This diameter should be checked by using a 10× measuring magnifier with graticule or a projection magnification.

FPOR

Only ANS give a tolerance of ±0.2 mm while stating that there is no appropriate measuring instrument available at the moment; however, a moiré fringe device could be used to estimate this parameter.

Edge lift

Only BS stipulate a tolerance, which is ±0.02 mm for both axial and radial edge lift. The recommended method of checking this parameter is to use the optical spherometer as described in Section 2.11, which was devised by Stone (1975).

Centration

Again only BS stipulate a tolerance, which is a maximum error of 0.5 mm, assessed using the focimeter.

Bifocal add

ANS and AS specify a tolerance of ±0.25 D on the addition, measured using a focimeter as for general BVP measurement.

Segment height

ANS and AS are in agreement on this parameter. The segment height tolerance is

+0.2 mm
−0.1 mm

BS stipulate a tolerance of

±0.1 mm

This is assessed using a 10× measuring magnifier or a projection magnification system.

6.7.2 Scleral lenses

A number of the tolerances imposed upon the corneal leans are also applied to the scleral lens.

BCOR
ANS and AS stipulate a tolerance of

±0.03 mm

BS stipulate

±0.05 mm

This can be checked with the optical spherometer, calibrated keratometer or by interferometry techniques.

BPOR
BS specify a tolerance of ±0.1 mm measured as for corneal lenses.

BPOD
BS stipulate a tolerance of ±0.2 mm measured as for corneal lenses.

Back scleral radius
BS and AS agree that the tolerance for this parameter should be ±0.1 mm measured as the BCOR.

BCOD
AS stipulate a tolerance of

±0.1 mm

BS stipulate

±0.2 mm

measured as for corneal lenses.

Basic or primary optic diameter
BS stipulate a tolerance of ±0.1 mm, to be assessed by the *sagitta* method described in Section 6.6.

OS (total diameter)
ANS and AS stipulate a tolerance of

±0.5 mm

BS stipulate

±0.25 mm

This is measured as for corneal lenses but not including the V gauge.

BVP
The tolerances are as for corneal lenses.

Prism
The tolerances are as for corneal lenses.

Cylinder power
The tolerances are as for corneal lenses.

Toric surface radii
The tolerances are as for corneal lenses.

Central thickness
There is universal agreement that the tolerance should be ±0.03 mm, measured as for corneal lenses.

FCOD
BS stipulate a tolerance of ±0.2 mm measured as for corneal lenses.

FCOR
ANS recommend a tolerance of ±0.02 mm measured as for corneal lenses.

Centration
BS specify a maximum error of 0.5 mm assessed using the focimeter.

Central clearance from cast
There is universal agreement that the tolerance should be ±0.02 mm measured by a dial gauge.

BS also stipulate that a 10% allowance on specification can be made for the fenestration, truncation, displacement, and haptic (scleral) thickness.

6.7.3 Soft lenses

BS recommend that soft lenses be tested at a temperature of 20±0.5°C hydrated in normal saline containing 9 g of sodium chloride per litre. Some of the tolerances apply to the dry lens and these are therefore probably of more interest to the contact lens manufacturer. ANS do not specify tolerances for soft lenses in Z80.2–1972.

BCOR
AS recommend ±0.05 mm for a hydrated lens. BS recommend ±0.1 mm for a dry lens, ±0.2 mm for a fully hydrated lens.

BPOR
Only BS stipulate a tolerance, at ±0.1 mm (dry) and ±0.2 mm (hydrated).

BCOD
Only BS stipulate a tolerance, at ±0.1 mm (dry).

BPOD
Only BS specify a tolerance, at ±0.2 mm (dry).

OS (total diameter)
AS specify a tolerance according to the water content of the material. Where this is less than 50% the tolerance is ±0.05 mm (hydrated). If the water content is above 50% then the tolerance is ±0.1 mm (hydrated).
   BS specify a tolerance of ±0.25 mm (hydrated).

BVP
AS and BS consider lens powers below and above 10 D and therefore stipulate two tolerances. In the case of AS these are ±0.12 D and ±0.25 D. BS stipulate ±0.25 D and ±0.50 D respectively. AS suggest that the lenses be blotted to remove surface moisture but not be allowed to dry for more than 15 s before a measurement is made.

Prism
AS stipulate ±0.25 Δ, BS stipulate ±0.50 Δ at the geometrical centre of the optic zone.

Cylinder power
BS specify the following tolerances:

for cylinder power up to 2.00 DC	±0.50 D	
for cylinder power of 2.00–4.00 DC	±0.75 D	hydrated
for cylinder power over 4.00 DC	±1.00 D	

Cylinder axis
AS and BS specify a tolerance of ±5°.

Central thickness
AS specify a tolerance of ±0.02 mm for a single lens and ±0.03 mm

for a pair of lenses. BS stipulate a tolerance of ±0.02 mm (dry) and ±0.05 mm (hydrated).

Edge thickness
BS stipulate a tolerance of ±0.02 mm (dry) and ±0.05 mm (hydrated).

FCOD
BS stipulate a tolerance of ±0.2 mm (dry) and ±0.2 mm (hydrated).

Centration
BS stipulate a maximum error of 0.5 mm.

6.8 Summary

The common tolerances discussed in this section are summarized in *Tables 6.1–6.3* above.

7 Computer programs

In the past any book dealing with the optics of contact lenses has been accompanied by sets of tables which allow the practitioner to arrive at the answer to particular problems quickly and conveniently. The author considered that, at a time when microcomputers are available at relatively small cost, it is more appropriate to replace tables with suitable simple computer programs. It is appreciated that many established optometrists may have little or no interest or ability in programming, and these people in particular will be able to see just how easy it is to organize a simple program using the computer language BASIC. A simple program which performs, for example, the effective power calculation can replace a number of pages of tables, and using such a program is more convenient than referring to tables.

The programs have been written so that each of them will run as an independent entity; however, there is a menu program which, if merged with all the preceding programs, provides the optometrist with a single menu-driven program that can be used to solve the common optics of contact lens problems encountered in clinical practice. A number of the programs provide the practitioner with information which allows a more precise assessment of the interrelationships encountered in fitting multicurve contact lenses to an aspheric cornea. Without this type of information the practitioner relies on his or her intuitive deductions and, after only a short time using programs like the ones included in this chapter, it becomes obvious that our intuitive conclusions often result in misleading deductions which lead to deteriorating rather than improved fitting relationships between the contact lens and the cornea. The program listings which follow were written for the Sinclair Spectrum computer; however, only minor modifications will produce a program that will run on other popular models.

The author is indebted to Jim Gilchrist, lecturer in optometry at Bradford University, for his help with the writing of these programs.

The following tests are available:

(1) Spectacle lens effective power at the cornea.
(2) Radius/power conversion in air.
(3) Radius/power conversion for an interface dividing media of any refractive index.
(4) Calculation of front vertex power and front surface radius.
(5) Calculation of peripheral radii required to give a specific axial edge lift for C2, C3 and C4 lenses.
(6) Calculation of the edge lift produced by any C2, C3 and C4 lenses.
(7) Calculation of peripheral radius required to give a specific axial edge lift in a contralateral offset bicurve lens.
(8) Calculation of x and p for an aspheric surface.
(9) Calculation of TLT and axial edge clearance for any C2, C3, C4, offset or aspheric lens.
(10) Calculation of junction and edge thickness in a lenticular.
(11) The power-to-radius conversion of the RC device.

The programs will now be examined individually. When the program is completed, type 'RUN' and enter this in order to activate the program.

7.1 Effective power (lines 1000–1160)

The effective power of a spectacle correction at the cornea is always required when, during an over-refraction, the lens in the refractor head or trial frame has a power greater than 4.00 D.

The program is very straightforward. Line 1010 clears the screen. Lines 1020–1070 print up the instructions and deal with the problem of acquiring the information. s is the power of the spectacle correction. v is the vertex distance. Lines 1080 and 1090 describe the step along method used for the calculation of effective power. Line 1100 rounds the effective power off to two decimal places. Line 1110 prints the answer on the screen. Lines 1120–1150 offer the option of repeating the exercise.

This simple program illustrates the fundamentals which are used throughout this chapter.

To use the program is simplicity itself. The computer asks for the power of the spectacle correction. When this is entered it asks for the vertex distance. When this is entered it prints the answer correct to two decimal places, and asks if you wish to repeat.

The listing is as follows.

```
1000 REM effect F
1010 CLS
1020 PRINT "EFFECTIVE POWER AT CORNEA."
1030 PRINT : PRINT : PRINT
1040 PRINT "enter power of spec. Rx (D)": INPUT s
1050 PRINT s;" dioptres."
1060 PRINT : PRINT "enter vertex distance (mm)": INPUT v
1070 PRINT v;" mm."
1080 LET s=1000/s
1090 LET ef=1000/(s-v)
1100 LET ef=INT (ef*100+.5)/100
1110 PRINT : PRINT "Effective power at cornea is
    ";ef;" D."
1120 PRINT : PRINT
1130 INPUT "Repeat?(y/n)";q$
1140 IF q$="y" THEN GO TO 1010
1150 IF q$="Y" THEN GO TO 1010
1160 RETURN
```

In order to check the program try the following:

(1) Power of spectacle R_x enter -12
    Vertex distance   enter 14
    This should give an effective power at the cornea of -10.27 D.

(2) Power of spectacle R_x enter 13
    Vertex distance   enter 14
    gives an effective power of $+15.89$ D.

7.2 Radius/power in air (lines 2000–2270)

The conversion of the radius of curvature to surface power or vice versa is a common clinical requirement which, when dealt with in tabular form, is restricted to a particular refractive index for each set of tables. The computer program has the advantage that it will deal with any refractive index. If the user enters 1.336 as the refractive index, then the program becomes a computerized version of Heine's scale.

Lines 2000–2090 once again print the instructions and acquire the information. Lines 2105–2130 perform the power-to-radius conversion. Line 2140 rounds the answer to two decimal places. Lines 2175–2200 perform a similar function for the radius-to-power conversion.

The program asks for the refractive index of the lens material. It then asks for the radius of curvature of the surface. If this is entered then the power of the surface is given in dioptres. If the user wishes to know the radius of curvature then the computer requests that '0' be entered. It then asks for the power of the surface and when this is entered it gives the radius of curvature required to produce the surface power. All answers are given to two decimal places. If the user wishes, for example, to acquire answers to three decimal places the lines 2140 and 2200 must be altered by changing the 100 to 1000 so that 2140, for example, would then read

LET r = INT(r*1000 + .5)/1000

The full listing of the program is given below.

```
2000 REM r/F
2010 CLS
2020 PRINT "Radius/power conversion in air."
2030 PRINT : PRINT
2040 PRINT "enter ref. index of medium": INPUT n
2050 PRINT n
2060 LET n=n*1000
2070 PRINT : PRINT "enter radius of surface OR"
2080 PRINT : PRINT "enter 0 if radius is required"
2090 INPUT r
2100 IF r<>0 THEN GO TO 2180
2105 REM power to radius conversion
2110 PRINT : PRINT "enter surface power in air (D)
    "
2120 INPUT f: PRINT f;" dioptres."
2130 LET r=(n-1000)/f
2140 LET r=INT (r*100+.5)/100
2150 IF r<0 THEN LET r=-r
2160 PRINT : PRINT "Radius of this surface is
    ";r;" mm."
2170 GO TO 2230
2175 REM radius to power conversion
2180 PRINT : PRINT r;" mm."
2190 LET f=(n-1000)/r
2200 LET f=INT (f*100+.5)/100
2210 PRINT : PRINT "Surface power is
        ";f;" D in air."
2220 PRINT : PRINT "(+ve for front surface -ve for
    back surface)"
2230 PRINT : PRINT
2240 INPUT "Repeat?(y/n)";q$
2250 IF q$="y" THEN GO TO 2010
2260 IF q$="Y" THEN GO TO 2010
2270 RETURN
```

In order to check the program try the following:

(1) Refractive index   enter 1.49
     Radius   enter 7.4
     This should give a surface power of 66.22 D.

(2) Refractive index   enter 1.336
     Radius   enter ∅
     Surface power   enter 43.64
     This should give a radius of curvature of 7.7 mm.

7.3 Interface radius/power conversion (lines 3000-3240)

This is of course a similar program to that of Section 7.2; however, the power or radius is given for any combination of refractive indices separated by the interface. Section 7.2 was designed with contact lenses specifically in mind where the front surface of the lens is always convex and the back surface is always concave so that the radii of curvature are always positive. This program, however, uses the sign convention in the usual way, assuming that medium 1 is to the left of medium 2 with light travelling from left to right.

This program is structured in a very similar way to that of Section 7.2. In using the program the computer asks for the refractive index of medium 1 and when this is entered it requests the refractive index of medium 2. As before you may now enter the interface radius to acquire its power or enter its power to acquire its radius.

The full listing of the program is given below.

```
3000 REM interface
3010 CLS
3020 PRINT "Radius/power at an interface."
3030 PRINT : PRINT
3040 PRINT "enter ref. index of medium 1.": PRINT
"(medium to left of interface)
": INPUT n1
3050 PRINT n1
3060 PRINT "enter ref. index of medium 2.": PRINT
"(medium to right of interface
)": INPUT n2
3070 PRINT n2
3080 LET n=(n2-n1)*1000
3090 PRINT : PRINT "enter radius of surface OR"
3100 PRINT : PRINT "enter 0 if radius is required"
```

```
3110 INPUT r
3115 IF r<>0 THEN PRINT "interface radius ",r;" mm
."
3120 IF r<>0 THEN GO TO 3180
3125 REM power/radius conversion
3130 PRINT : PRINT "enter interface power (D)"
3140 INPUT f: PRINT f;" dioptres."
3150 LET r=INT ((n/f)*100+.5)/100
3160 PRINT : PRINT "Interface radius is ",r;" mm."
3170 GO TO 3200
3175 REM radius/power conversion
3180 LET f=INT ((n/r)*100+.5)/100
3190 PRINT : PRINT "Interface power is",f;" dioptr
es."
3200 PRINT : PRINT
3210 INPUT "Repeat (y/n)";q$
3220 IF q$="y" THEN GO TO 3010
3230 IF q$="Y" THEN GO TO 3010
3240 RETURN
```

In order to check the program try the following:

(1) Refractive index of medium 1   enter 1.49
    Refractive index of medium 2   enter 1.336
    Radius   enter 7.8
    This should give an interface power of -19.74 D.

(2) Repeat the above but enter ∅ for the radius; then
    Interface power   enter -19.74
    This should give an interface radius of 7.8 mm.

7.4 Front surface radius and FVP (lines 4000–4260)

This program calculates the front surface radius and FVP of a contact lens, given the BVP; central thickness; BCOR; and refractive index. This is of course what the manufacturer needs to know when producing a lens with a BVP equal to that requested by the optometrist. It may be useful to the practitioner in that it gives an immediate indication of the relationship between the front and back surfaces of the contact lens. Lines 4120–4190 perform the calculations, and upon examination the reader will see that we are asking the computer to use the step along method to acquire the answers.

In using the program the computer requests the user to enter the lens BVP, followed by the centre thickness; the BCOR; and finally

Front surface radius and FVP (lines 4000-4260)

the refractive index. The computer immediately indicates the front vertex power and the front surface radius, both to two decimal places.

The full listing of the program is given below.

```
4000 REM FVP r1
4010 CLS
4020 PRINT "Front surface radius and FVP."
4030 PRINT : PRINT
4040 PRINT "enter BVP (D)": INPUT b
4050 PRINT b;" dioptres."
4060 PRINT : PRINT "enter lens centre thickness (m
m)": INPUT t
4070 PRINT t;" mm."
4080 PRINT : PRINT "enter B.C.O.R. (mm)": INPUT r2
4090 PRINT r2;" mm."
4100 PRINT : PRINT "enter ref. -index": INPUT n
4110 PRINT n
4120 LET f2=(1-n)*1000/r2
4130 LET t=t/1000: LET f1=b-f2: LET f1=1/f1
4140 LET f1=f1+t/n: LET f1=1/f1
4150 LET r1=(n-1)*1000/f1
4160 LET f=1/f2: LET f=f-t/n
4170 LET f=1/f: LET f=f+f1
4180 LET f=INT (f*100+.5)/100
4190 LET r1=INT (r1*100+.5)/100
4200 PRINT : PRINT "Front vertex power is
    ";f;" dioptres."
4210 PRINT : PRINT "Front surface radius is
    ";r1;" mm."
4220 PRINT : PRINT
4230 INPUT "Repeat?(y/n)";q$
4240 IF q$="y" THEN GO TO 4010
4250 IF q$="Y" THEN GO TO 4010
4260 RETURN
```

In order to check the program try the following:

BVP	enter 5.5
Lens centre thickness	enter .6
BCOR	enter 7.8
Refractive index	enter 1.49

This should give a front vertex power of 5.22 D and a front surface radius of 7.37 mm.

7.5 Axial edge lift (lines 5000–5910)

This program calculates the BPORs required for any C2, C3 or C4 lens to give a stipulated axial edge lift. In the case of the C2 lens the single peripheral curve produces all the edge lift. The two peripheral curves in the C3 share the edge lift, with the mid-curve producing two-thirds and the outer curve one-third of the total edge lift. In the case of the C4, the first peripheral curve is responsible for generating half of the total edge lift, with the second peripheral curve generating one-third and the final outer curve one-sixth of the total edge lift. The instructions are given in lines 5145–5170. Originally the program was written to share the edge lift equally between the curves but this was found to produce a lens design which often possessed a very flat peripheral curve for the C3 and C4 lenses. The modified edge lift sharing described above produces lenses very similar to those described and used by Stone (1975) and Rabbetts (1976).

If the practitioner wished to perform this exercise without a computer, then it would be necessary to use an iterative technique substituting likely values into the equations and repeating the calculations until the stipulated edge lift is achieved. This program instructs the computer to do exactly the same thing and it can take it some time to find the appropriate radii. The request to repeat the calculations is made by setting up a FOR–NEXT loop which the computer will circumnavigate repeatedly until an appropriate radius is found. Lines 5700–5900 contain the FOR–NEXT loop which performs the radius searches. This commences with a rapid search which acquires an approximate radius quickly whereupon the computer re-enters the loop in order to determine an accurate radius. Line 5715 is an instruction peculiar to the Sinclair Spectrum and it is there simply to sound a short high pitched note every time the computer tries a new radius value. It can therefore be ignored when programming any other computer.

In using the program the computer first asks how many back surface curves the lens has. It then asks the user to enter the axial edge lift. This is followed by requests for the BCOR; BCOD; and the diameter for the axial edge lift. The computer then enters the FOR–NEXT loop in order to find the BPORs that give the stipulated axial edge lift. The precision of the axial edge lift will determine how many radii fulfil the requirement. This program prints out all radii that will give the axial edge lift requested, plus or minus a maximum error of 0.002 mm. If the list is a long one the Spectrum computer may print 'scroll'. If this happens press the 'y' key to complete the list. The user then needs to select and enter a radius from the list and should select a convenient radius from the middle region of the list where this is lengthy. If the lens is a bicurve then the program ends by printing the lens specification. If the lens is a C3 or C4 the computer asks the user to enter BPOD.1, and after a short wait a list of radius values for the second peripheral curve will be displayed and again the user must select a suitable radius. The program ends by displaying the lens specification if a C3 is being considered. If the lens is a C4 the user is asked to enter BPOD.2 and this results in the final list of radii appearing on the screen with a request to select a suitable value. This results in the specification of the C4 being displayed on the screen.

The full listing of the program is given below.

```
5000 REM AEL=r
5005 DIM r(10): DIM d(10): DIM z(10)
5010 CLS
5020 PRINT "AXIAL EDGE LIFT.": PRINT
5030 PRINT "This computes the B.P.O.R.s"
5040 PRINT "to give any desired AEL for any"
5050 PRINT "C2,C3, or C4 lens.": PRINT
5080 PRINT "How many back surface curves?": INPUT c
5090 PRINT "C";c;" lens"
5100 IF c<2 THEN PRINT "NOT AVAILABLE": PAUSE 100: CLS : GO TO 5080
5110 IF c>4 THEN PRINT "NOT AVAILABLE": PAUSE 100: CLS : GO TO 5080
5120 FOR i=1 TO c
5125 LET r(i)=0: LET d(i)=0: REM initialise curve parameters
5130 NEXT i
5135 PRINT "enter axial edge lift required": INPUT z
5140 PRINT z;" mm."
5145 IF c=2 THEN LET z(1)=INT (z*1000+.5)/1000
5150 IF c=3 THEN LET z(1)=INT ((2*z/3)*1000+.5)/1000
5155 IF c=3 THEN LET z(2)=INT ((z/3)*1000+.5)/1000
5160 IF c=4 THEN LET z(1)=INT ((z/2)*1000+.5)/1000
5165 IF c=4 THEN LET z(2)=INT ((z/3)*1000+.5)/1000
5170 IF c=4 THEN LET z(3)=INT ((z/6)*1000+.5)/1000
5180 REM input central curve parameters
5190 PRINT "enter B.C.O.R.": INPUT r(1): PRINT r(1);" mm."
5200 PRINT "enter B.C.O.D.": INPUT d(1): PRINT d(1);" mm."
5210 PRINT "enter diameter for edge lift": INPUT d(c)
5220 PRINT d(c);" mm.": REM this assumes AEL at overall diameter
```

Computer programs

```
5230 REM determine peripheral curve diameters
5240 FOR i=2 TO c
5250 CLS : PRINT : PRINT "PLEASE WAIT"
5260 PRINT "Computing the peripheral curves"
5270 LET y1=d(i-1)/2: LET y2=d(c)/2
5280 LET sf=0: REM flag to indicate quick search
5290 LET ba=r(1)*100: LET st=20: REM quick search
parameters
5300 GO SUB 5700: REM quick radius search
5310 LET sf=1: REM flag for full radius search
5320 IF i=2 THEN LET ba=(q)*100: LET st=1
5330 IF i=3 THEN LET ba=(q)*100: LET st=2
5340 IF i=4 THEN LET ba=(q+1)*100: LET st=5
5350 GO SUB 5700: REM full radius search
5360 PRINT "These are the peripheral radii"
5370 PRINT : PRINT "select B.P.O.R.";i-1: INPUT r(
i): PRINT r(i);" mm."
5380 IF i<>c THEN PRINT "enter the B.P.O.D.";i-1:
INPUT d(i)
5390 NEXT i
5400 REM deliver specification
5410 PRINT : PRINT "The back surface specification
"
5420 PRINT "is        C";c
5430 PRINT "B.C.O.R. ",r(1),"B.C.O.D. ",d(1)
5440 FOR i=2 TO c
5450 PRINT "B.P.O.R.";i-1,r(i),"B.P.O.D.";i-1,d(i)
5460 NEXT i
5470 PRINT : PRINT "for axial edge lift of ";z;" m
m."
5480 PRINT : PRINT "at diameter of ";d(c);" mm."
5490 PRINT : INPUT "REPEAT?(y/n)";q$
5500 IF q$="y" THEN GO TO 5010
5510 IF q$="Y" THEN GO TO 5010
5520 GO TO 10
5700 REM radius search routine
5710 FOR j=ba TO 9000 STEP st
5715 BEEP .01,50
5720 LET r2=j/100
5730 LET a=r(i-1)-SQR ((r(i-1)*r(i-1))-(y2*y2))
5740 LET s1=r(i-1)-SQR ((r(i-1)*r(i-1))-(y1*y1))
5750 LET s2=r2-SQR ((r2*r2)-(y2*y2))
5760 LET s3=r2-SQR ((r2*r2)-(y1*y1))
5770 LET p=s1+s2-s3
5780 LET e=INT ((a-p)*1000+.5)/1000
5790 IF sf=1 THEN GO TO 5850
5800 REM the quick search
5810 LET e=INT (e*10+.5)/10
5820 LET u=INT (z(i-1)*10+.5)/10
5830 IF e>=u THEN LET q=r2: GO TO 5910
```

```
5840 GO TO 5900
5850 REM the radius search
5860 IF e=z(i-1)-.001 THEN PRINT INT (r2*100+.5)/1
00
5870 IF e=z(i-1) THEN PRINT INT (r2*100+.5)/100
5880 IF e=z(i-1)+.001 THEN PRINT INT (r2*100+.5)/1
00
5890 IF e>z(i-1)+.001 THEN GO TO 5910
5900 NEXT j
5910 RETURN
```

In order to check the program try the following:

(1) C2
Back surface curves   enter 2
Axial edge lift   enter .14
BCOR   enter 7.8
BCOD   enter 6.5
Diameter for edge lift   enter 8.5
This should give BPORs of 9.87–9.92 mm.
Select BPOR   enter 9.9
and the full specification should be displayed.

(2) C3
Back surface curves   enter 3
Axial edge lift   enter .12
BCOR   enter 7
BCOD   enter 7
Diameter for edge lift   enter 8.6
This should give BPOR.1s of 7.84–7.87 mm.
Select BPOR.1   enter 7.85
Select BPOD.1   enter 7.8
This should give BPOR.2s of 8.94–9.02 mm.
Select BPOR.2   enter 9
and the full specification should be displayed.

(3) C4
Back surface curves   enter 4
Axial edge lift   enter .15
BCOR   enter 8.6
BCOD   enter 7
Diameter for edge lift   enter 9.2
This should give BPOR.1s of 9.57–9.6 mm.
Select BPOR.1   enter 9.6
Select BPOD.1   enter 7.8
This should give BPOR.2s of 10.92–10.96 mm.
Select BPOR.2   enter 10.95

Select BPOD.2   enter 8.60
This should give BPOR.3s of 12.95–13.1 mm.
Select BPOR.3   enter 13
and the full specification should be displayed.

7.6 Edge thickness and edge lift (lines 6000–6650)

This program represents an alternative and more flexible approach to the problem of edge lift. The user simply enters the lens specification and the computer calculates the edge lift. The previous program (Section 7.5) can be used to determine some suitable radii from which to start. These radii can then be altered and the effect of the alterations on the axial edge lift will be immediately seen. This program also gives the radial edge lift (radial to the back central optic), and can be used to give the axial edge thickness where the lens power and central thickness are known. The program is designed to work for C2, C3, C4, offset and aspheric lenses although in the latter two types the program requests the axial edge lift and calculates the radial edge lift.

The user is first asked if the lens is an offset or aspheric. If 'n' is entered then the computer requests the lens BCOR and BCOD and then asks how many curves the lens has. This is followed by requests for the peripheral curve radii and diameters. The final diameter must be the diameter for the axial edge lift. The computer then asks if the user requires lens thickness information. Where this is required the computer requests the lens BVP, central thickness and refractive index. This results in the computer calculating the front surface radius; the front surface power; and the axial edge thickness. The computer also displays the axial and radial edge lift (radial to the central back surface curve). These latter two features are displayed alone where no request for thickness information is made. If the user enters 'y' for the offset/aspheric option then the computer requests the BCOR; the diameter for the edge lift; (BVP; centre thickness; and refractive index where edge thickness information is requested) and the axial edge lift. This results in the display of front surface radius; front surface power; axial edge thickness; radial edge thickness where the BVP, centre thickness, and refractive index have been entered; and the radial edge lift. All answers in this program are given to three decimal places.

The full listing of the program is given below.

```
6000 REM r=AEL
6005 DIM r(10): DIM d(10)
6010 CLS
6020 PRINT : PRINT "COMPUTATION OF EDGE LIFT AND"
6025 PRINT "THICKNESS."
6030 PRINT : PRINT "This section computes edge lif
t"
6040 PRINT "and thickness from the lens"
6050 PRINT "parameters for C2,C3 and C4 "
6055 PRINT "lenses"
6060 PRINT "It also computes the radial  "
6070 PRINT "edge spec. for OFFSET and"
6075 PRINT "ASPHERIC lenses."
6080 LET lf=0: REM reset lens flag
6090 PRINT : PRINT "Offset or Aspheric?(y/n)": INP
UT q$
6100 IF q$="Y" THEN LET lf=1
6110 IF q$="y" THEN LET lf=1
6115 PRINT : PRINT "enter BCOR": INPUT r(1): PRINT
 r(1);" mm."
6120 IF lf=1 THEN GO TO 6200
6125 REM multicurve data input
6130 PRINT "enter BCOD": INPUT d(1): PRINT d(1);"
mm."
6140 PRINT : PRINT "How many curves?": INPUT c
6150 IF c<2 THEN PRINT "NOT AVAILABLE": GO TO 6140
6155 IF c>4 THEN PRINT "NOT AVAILABLE": GO TO 6140
6160 FOR i=2 TO c
6165 PRINT "enter": PRINT "BPOR";i-1;"          B
POD";i-1: INPUT r(i),d(i): PRI
NT r(i),d(i)
6170 NEXT i
6175 IF c=2 THEN LET y=d(2)
6180 IF c=3 THEN LET y=d(3)
6185 IF c=4 THEN LET y=d(4)
6190 PRINT "          This is the diameter"
6195 PRINT "               for the AEL."
6200 IF lf=1 THEN PRINT "enter diameter for edge l
ift.": INPUT y: PRINT y;" mm."
6215 PRINT : PRINT "Do you want lens thickness ":
PRINT "information?(y/n)": INP
UT e$
6220 IF e$="n" THEN GO TO 6240
6225 PRINT : PRINT "enter BVP (dioptres)": INPUT p
: PRINT p;" D."
6230 PRINT "enter centre thickness (mm)": INPUT t:
 PRINT t;" mm."
6235 PRINT "enter refractive index": INPUT n: PRIN
T n
```

```
6240 IF lf=1 THEN PRINT : PRINT "enter axial edge
lift": INPUT z: PRINT z;" mm."
6245 IF e$="n" THEN GO TO 6340
6250 REM front surface radius and FVP
6260 LET f2=(1-n)*1000/r(1)
6270 LET f1=1000/((1000/(p-f2))+(t/n))
6280 LET rf=(n-1)*1000/f1
6290 LET f1=INT (f1*100+.5)/100
6300 LET rf=INT (rf*100+.5)/100
6310 PRINT : PRINT "Front surface radius is",rf;"
mm."
6320 PRINT "Front surface power is",f1;" D."
6330 LET s1=rf-SQR (rf*rf-(y/2)*(y/2))
6340 LET s2=r(1)-SQR (r(1)*r(1)-(y/2)*(y/2))
6350 IF lf=1 THEN GO TO 6510
6355 REM compute multicurve edge parameters
6360 LET o=0
6370 LET so=r(1)-SQR (r(1)*r(1)-d(1)/2*(d(1)/2))
6380 FOR i=2 TO c
6390 LET s3=r(i)-SQR (r(i)*r(i)-(d(i)/2)*(d(i)/2))
6400 LET s4=r(i)-SQR (r(i)*r(i)-(d(i-1)/2)*(d(i-1)
/2))
6410 LET o=o+s3-s4
6420 NEXT i
6430 LET o=o+so
6435 IF e$="n" THEN GO TO 6450
6440 LET te=INT ((o-s1+t)*1000+.5)/1000
6450 LET z=INT ((s2-o)*1000+.5)/1000
6460 LET e=SQR ((r(1)-o)*(r(1)-o)+(y/2*y/2))-r(1)
6470 LET e=INT (e*1000+.5)/1000
6475 IF e$="n" THEN GO TO 6490
6480 PRINT : PRINT "axial edge thickness at ";y;"
mm. is ",te;" mm."
6490 PRINT "axial edge lift at ";y;" mm. is ",z;"
mm."
6500 PRINT "radial edge lift at ";y;" mm. is ",e;"
 mm."
6505 GO TO 6620
6510 REM offset and aspheric
6515 IF e$="n" THEN GO TO 6530
6520 LET te=s2-s1-z+t
6530 LET rr=s2-z: LET rr=r(1)-rr
6540 LET e=SQR ((rr*rr)+(y/2*y/2))-r(1)
6550 LET e=INT (e*1000+.5)/1000
6555 IF e$="n" THEN GO TO 6610
6560 LET rv=ATN (y/(2*(rf-te-s1)))
6570 LET tr=rf-(y/(2*SIN (rv)))
6580 LET tr=INT (tr*1000+.5)/1000
6585 LET te=INT (te*1000+.5)/1000
```

Edge thickness and edge lift (lines 6000-6650)   189

```
6590 PRINT : PRINT "axial edge thickness at ";y;"
mm. is ",te;" mm."
6600 PRINT "radial edge thickness at ";y;" mm. is
";tr;" mm."
6610 PRINT "radial edge lift at ";y;" mm. is ",e;"
 mm."
6615 REM ---------------------------
6620 PRINT : INPUT "REPEAT?(y/n)";q$
6630 IF q$="Y" THEN GO TO 6010
6640 IF q$="y" THEN GO TO 6010
6650 RETURN
```

In order to check the program try the following:

(1)   Offset or aspheric   enter n
     BCOR   enter 7.8
     BCOD   enter 6.5
     How many curves   enter 2
     BPOR.1   enter 9.9
     BPOD.1   enter 8.6
     Lens thickness information   enter n
     This should give an axial edge lift of 0.149 mm, with a radial edge lift of 0.125 mm.

(2)   Offset or aspheric   enter n
     BCOR   enter 7
     BCOD   enter 7
     How many curves   enter 3
     BPOR.1   enter 7.85
     BPOD.1   enter 7.8
     BPOR.2   enter 9
     BPOD.2   enter 8.6
     Lens thickness information   enter n
     This should give an axial edge lift of 0.12 mm, with a radial edge lift of 0.095 mm.

(3)   Offset or aspheric   enter n
     BCOR   enter 9
     BCOD   enter 7.5
     How many curves   enter 4
     BPOR.1   enter 10.55
     BPOD.1   enter 8.2
     BPOR.2   enter 12.85
     BPOD.2   enter 9
     BPOR.3   enter 15.25

BPOD.3 enter 9.5
Lens thickness information enter y
BVP enter −6
Centre thickness enter .3
Refractive index enter 1.49
This should result in a display which indicates:
Front surface radius 10.21 mm
Front surface power 47.98 D
Axial edge thickness 0.308 mm
Axial edge lift 0.175 mm
Radial edge lift 0.149 mm

(4) Offset or aspheric enter y
BCOR enter 7.2
Diameter for edge lift enter 9.5
Lens thickness information enter y
BVP enter −6
Centre thickness enter .3
Refractive index enter 1.49
Axial edge lift enter .12
This should give the following:
Front surface radius 7.99 mm
Front surface power 61.29 D
Axial edge thickness 0.404 mm
Radial edge thickness 0.321 mm
Radial edge lift 0.091 mm

7.7 BPOR for an offset lens (lines 7000–7300)

This program calculates the BPOR required for a contralateral offset bicurve lens to give any requested axial edge lift. The program is similar to that of Section 7.5 in that it uses a FOR–NEXT loop in order to conduct a series of iterative calculations until the requested edge lift is achieved. This loop runs from line 7110 to 7230. Once again the computer prints radii that induce the requested edge lift, plus or minus a maximum error of 0.002 mm.

The user is asked to enter the axial edge lift required, followed by the BCOR; BCOD; and the diameter for the edge lift. As before, line 7115 instructs the computer to make a short high pitched note each time it re-enters the loop. The radii which induce the edge lift to within 0.002 mm are listed on the screen followed by the option to repeat if required.

The full listing of the program is given below.

```
7000 REM EL2
7010 CLS
7020 PRINT "PERIPHERAL RADIUS OF"
7025 PRINT "OFFSET LENS."
7030 PRINT : PRINT "This section computes the BPOR
"
7040 PRINT "required to give any desired "
7050 PRINT "axial edge lift on an offset"
7055 PRINT "bicurve lens."
7060 PRINT : PRINT "enter axial edge lift": INPUT
 z: PRINT z;" mm."
7070 PRINT "enter BCOR ": INPUT r: PRINT r;" mm."
7080 PRINT "enter BCOD ": INPUT d: PRINT d;" mm."
7090 PRINT "enter diameter for edge lift": INPUT y
: PRINT y;" mm.": PRINT
7095 PRINT "PLEASE WAIT."
7100 REM search for radius
7105 LET z=INT (z*100+.5)/100
7110 FOR i=(r+(z*40))*100 TO 9000 STEP 10
7115 BEEP .01,50
7120 LET r1=i/100
7130 LET y1=(d/2)+((d/(2*r))*(r1-r))
7140 LET y2=(y/2)+((d/(2*r))*(r1-r))
7150 LET s1=r-SQR (r*r-(d/2)*(d/2))
7160 LET s2=r-SQR (r*r-(y/2)*(y/2))
7170 LET s3=r1-SQR (r1*r1-y1*y1)
7180 LET s4=r1-SQR (r1*r1-y2*y2)
7190 LET e=(s2-s1)-(s4-s3)
7200 LET e=INT (e*500+.5)/500
7210 IF e=z THEN PRINT r1
7220 IF e>z THEN GO TO 7240
7230 NEXT i
7240 PRINT : PRINT "These are the required ": PRIN
T "BPOR values"
7250 PRINT : PRINT "for axial edge lift of";z;" mm
."
7260 PRINT : PRINT "at a diameter of ";y;" mm."
7270 PRINT : PRINT "REPEAT?(y/n)": INPUT q$
7280 IF q$="y" THEN GO TO 7010
7290 IF q$="Y" THEN GO TO 7010
7300 RETURN
```

In order to check the program try the following:

Axial edge lift	enter .12
BCOR	enter 7.2
BCOD	enter 6.5
Diameter for edge lift	enter 9.5

This should result in BPORs of 12.6–12.7 mm.

7.8 Aspheric surfaces (lines 8000–8230)

This program calculates the *p* value and the primary sag *x* of a conicoid surface.

The user is asked to indicate the central vertex radius followed by the diameter and the axial edge lift at this diameter. The computer then displays the *x* and *p* values to three decimal places.

The user is reminded on the screen that the *x* value can be checked on an aspheric lens by using the optical spherometer as described in Section 2.11.

The complete listing of the program is given below.

```
8000 REM aspheric
8010 CLS
8020 PRINT : PRINT "ASPHERIC SURFACE"
8030 PRINT : PRINT "This section computes x and p"
8040 PRINT "for an aspheric surface."
8050 PRINT : PRINT "enter central vertex radius": INPUT r: PRINT r;" mm."
8060 PRINT "enter diameter": INPUT d: PRINT d;" mm."
8070 PRINT "enter axial edge lift": INPUT z: PRINT z;" mm."
8080 LET s=r-SQR (r*r-(d/2)*(d/2))
8090 LET x=s-z
8100 LET p=((2*r*x)-(d/2*d/2))/(x*x)
8120 LET x=INT (x*1000+.5)/1000
8130 LET p=INT (p*1000+.5)/1000
8140 PRINT : PRINT "The x value for this lens is ",x;" mm."
8150 PRINT "This is the primary sag which": PRINT "may be checked on the optical ": PRINT "spherometer."
8160 PRINT : PRINT "The p value for this lens is",p
8165 PRINT "p<0 indicates a hyperboloid"
8170 PRINT "p=0 indicates a paraboloid"
8180 PRINT "p>0 indicates an ellipsoid"
8190 PRINT "p=1 indicates a sphere"
8200 PRINT : PRINT "REPEAT?(y/n)": INPUT q$
8210 IF q$="y" THEN GO TO 8010
8220 IF q$="Y" THEN GO TO 8010
8230 RETURN
```

In order to check the program try the following:

Central vertex radius	enter 7.85
Diameter	enter 9.5

Axial edge lift	enter .12

This should result in:

x value	1.48 mm
p value	0.309

7.9 TLT and axial edge clearance (lines 8600–9990)

This program will calculate the tear layer thickness at the corneal vertex and the axial edge clearance from the cornea at a specified diameter for a C2, C3, C4, contralateral offset bicurve or aspheric contact lens. The program uses a FOR–NEXT loop and calculates sags for progressively increasing diameters for both the cornea and the contact lens. If the sag of the contact lens is larger than that of the cornea then clearly the lens apex will be lifted off the corneal apex and the TLT will be greater than zero. The program compares the increase in sag from one diameter to the next, and providing that the increase in sag of the contact lens is greater than that of the cornea then the TLT will continue to increase. When this situation reverses and the increase in sag of the cornea is the greater then the contact ring has been determined. For the C2, C3 and C4 lenses (if fitted steep) this diameter is equal to the BCOD. For a toric cornea the program can only be applied to the flat meridian and the contact diameter will refer to the diameter along this meridian only. Where lenses are fitted flat in relation to the cornea the TLT has a value of zero as does the contact diameter.

The user is asked to enter the corneal radius followed by a request for the p value of the cornea. If this is not known an average value of 0.8 can be entered. The computer then asks if the lens is an aspheric or an offset bicurve. The user is then asked to enter the contact lens back surface parameters. Surplus parameters are entered as zero. Finally the user is asked to enter the diameter for the edge clearance. The computer may require some time before it displays the TLT, the contact diameter, the axial edge clearance and the primary sag of the cornea (all to three decimal places). This is followed by an option to repeat the exercise on the same cornea using a different contact lens. If this option is rejected then it is replaced by an option to repeat the exercise using different corneal parameters.

The program can be used to analyse what happens on a toric cornea with a little extra arithmetic. The user should determine the axial edge clearance along the flat meridian and also note the primary sag of the cornea for his meridian. A repeat run should then be requested for another cornea in order to determine the primary sag of the steep corneal meridian.

Enter the new corneal radius and the *p* value, and then reject the options for the aspheric and the offset lenses. The computer will then request the contact lense back surface radii and diameters. Enter zero for all of these but be sure to enter the correct diameter when the computer requests 'Enter diameter for edge clearance'. The program will give the TLT, contact diameter, axial edge clearance, and the primary sag of the cornea. Only the latter dimension has now any relevance.

The axial edge clearance on the steep corneal meridian can now be easily calculated by subtracting the flat primary sag from the steep primary sag of the cornea and adding this result to the axial edge clearance of the flat meridian. The difference between the two corneal primary sags indicates the extra edge clearance induced by the steeper corneal curve, and if this is added to the edge clearance for the flat meridian it obviously indicates the axial edge clearance for the steeper corneal meridian.

The full listing of the program is given below.

```
8600 REM TLT EC
8610 CLS
8620 PRINT "TLT and AXIAL EDGE CLEARANCE.": PRINT
8630 PRINT "This program will run for C2 C3": PRIN
T "C4 offset & aspheric lenses
.": PRINT : PRINT "ENTER 0 FOR SURPLUS PARAMETERS.
"
8640 PRINT : PRINT "Enter corneal radius.": INPUT
ro: PRINT ro;" mm."
8650 LET ro=ro*20
8660 PRINT "Enter p value for cornea.": INPUT p: P
RINT p
8670 GO SUB 9020
8680 LET ps=0: LET px=0
8685 CLS : PRINT "COMPUTING NOW."
8690 FOR y=1 TO yt
8700 IF y<=y1 THEN LET s=r1-SQR (r1*r1-y*y)
8710 IF y>y1 AND y<=y2 THEN LET s=(r1-SQR (r1*r1-y
1*y1))+(r2-SQR (r2*r2-y*y))-(r
2-SQR (r2*r2-y1*y1))
8720 IF y>y2 AND y<=y3 THEN LET s=(r1-SQR (r1*r1-y
1*y1))+(r2-SQR (r2*r2-y2*y2))-
(r2-SQR (r2*r2-y1*y1))+(r3-SQR (r3*r3-y*y))-(r3-SQ
R (r3*r3-y2*y2))
8730 IF y>y3 AND y<=y4 THEN LET s=(r1-SQR (r1*r1-y
1*y1))+(r2-SQR (r2*r2-y2*y2))-
```

TLT and axial edge clearance (lines 8600–9990)

```
(r2-SQR (r2*r2-y1*y1))+(r3-SQR (r3*r3-y3*y3))-(r3-
SQR (r3*r3-y2*y2))+(r4-SQR (r4
*r4-y*y))-(r4-SQR (r4*r4-y3*y3))
8740 LET dif=s-ps
8750 LET rr=ro/p
8760 LET x=rr-SQR (rr*rr-(y*y)/p)
8770 LET dif2=x-px
8780 IF dif2>(dif+.0001) THEN LET tlt=ps-px: LET y
c=y-1: GO TO 8830
8790 LET ps=s: LET px=x
8800 BEEP .01,50
8810 NEXT y
8820 LET tlt=ps-px: LET yc=y-1
8830 IF tlt<=0 THEN LET tlt=0: LET y=0: LET yc=0
8840 LET tlt=tlt/20: LET tlt=INT (tlt*1000+.5)/100
0
8850 PRINT : PRINT "TLT = ";tlt;" mm.": PRINT : PR
INT "CONTACT DIAMETER = ";yc/1
0;" mm.": PRINT
8860 IF yt>y1 AND yt<=y2 THEN LET s=(r1-SQR (r1*r1
-y1*y1))+(r2-SQR (r2*r2-yt*yt)
)-(r2-SQR (r2*r2-y1*y1))
8870 IF yt>y2 AND yt<=y3 THEN LET s=(r1-SQR (r1*r1
-y1*y1))+(r2-SQR (r2*r2-y2*y2)
)-(r2-SQR (r2*r2-y1*y1))+(r3-SQR (r3*r3-yt*yt))-(r
3-SQR (r3*r3-y2*y2))
8880 IF yt>y3 AND yt<=y4 THEN LET s=(r1-SQR (r1*r1
-y1*y1))+(r2-SQR (r2*r2-y2*y2)
)-(r2-SQR (r2*r2-y1*y1))+(r3-SQR (r3*r3-y3*y3))-(r
3-SQR (r3*r3-y2*y2))+(r4-SQR (
r4*r4-yt*yt))-(r4-SQR (r4*r4-y3*y3))
8890 LET rr=ro/p: LET x=rr-SQR (rr*rr-(yt*yt)/p)
8900 LET x=x/20: LET s=s/20
8910 LET ec=tlt+x-s
8920 LET ec=INT (ec*1000+.5)/1000: LET x=INT (x*10
00+.5)/1000
8930 PRINT "AXIAL EDGE CLEARANCE = ";ec;" mm.": PR
INT "at diameter ";yt/10;" mm.
"
8940 PRINT : PRINT "Prim. sag of cornea = ";x;" mm
."
8950 PRINT : PRINT "Do you have another lens for":
 PRINT "this cornea? y/n.": I
NPUT q$
8960 IF q$="y" THEN GO TO 8670
8970 IF q$="Y" THEN GO TO 8670
8980 PRINT : PRINT "Do you wish to examine another
": PRINT "cornea? y/n.": INPU
T q$
8990 IF q$="y" THEN GO TO 8610
```

Computer programs

```
9000 IF q$="Y" THEN GO TO 8610
9010 RETURN
9020 PRINT : PRINT "Is the lens an aspheric?  y/n.
": PRINT : INPUT q$
9030 IF q$="y" THEN GO TO 9700
9040 IF q$="Y" THEN GO TO 9700
9050 PRINT : PRINT "Is the lens an offset bicurve?
": PRINT "            y/n.":
 INPUT r$
9060 IF r$="y" THEN GO TO 9090
9070 IF r$="Y" THEN GO TO 9090
9075 GO TO 9540
9080 REM offset
9090 PRINT "Enter BCOR.    BCOD.": INPUT r1,y1: P
RINT "         ";r1;" mm.",y1;" m
m."
9100 PRINT "Enter axial edge lift.": INPUT z: PRIN
T z;" mm."
9110 PRINT "Enter diameter for edge lift.": INPUT
yt: PRINT yt;" mm."
9120 LET z=INT (z*1000+.5)/1000
9130 CLS : PRINT "COMPUTING THE BPOR."
9140 FOR i=r1*140 TO 6000 STEP 5
9150 BEEP .05,55
9160 LET r2=i/100
9170 LET s1=r1-SQR (r1*r1-(y1/2*y1/2))
9180 LET s2=r1-SQR (r1*r1-(yt/2*yt/2))
9190 LET yy=(y1/2)/r1*(r2-r1)
9200 LET y2=y1/2+yy: LET y3=yt/2+yy
9210 LET s3=r2-SQR (r2*r2-y2*y2)
9220 LET s4=r2-SQR (r2*r2-y3*y3)
9230 LET e=(s2-s1)-(s4-s3): LET e=INT (e*1000+.5)/
1000
9240 IF e=z THEN PRINT r2
9250 IF e>z THEN GO TO 9270
9260 NEXT i
9270 PRINT "These are the BPORs for the": PRINT "r
equired edge lift."
9280 PRINT : PRINT "Select a suitable BPOR.": INPU
T r2
9290 PRINT r2;" mm."
9300 LET yt=yt*10: LET z=z*20: LET y1=y1*10: LET r
1=r1*20: LET r2=r2*20
9310 REM lens equation
9320 LET x1=r1-SQR (r1*r1-yt*yt)-z
9330 REM corneal equation
9340 LET rr=ro/p
9350 LET xct=rr-SQR (rr*rr-(yt*yt)/p)
9360 REM loop for sags
9370 REM contact lens
```

```
9380 LET ps=0: LET px=0
9385 CLS : PRINT "COMPUTING NOW."
9390 FOR y=1 TO yt
9400 IF y<=y1 THEN LET s=r1-SQR (r1*r1-y*y)
9410 LET o=(r2-r1)*y1/r1
9420 IF y>y1 THEN LET s=(r1-SQR (r1*r1-y1*y1))+(r2
-SQR (r2*r2-(y+o)*(y+o)))-(r2-
SQR (r2*r2-(y1+o)*(y1+o)))
9430 LET dif=s-ps
9440 LET rr=ro/p
9450 LET x=rr-SQR (rr*rr-(y*y)/p)
9460 LET dif2=x-px
9470 IF dif2>(dif+.0001) THEN LET tlt=ps-px: LET y
c=y-1: GO TO 9920
9480 LET ps=s: LET px=x
9490 BEEP .01,50
9500 NEXT y
9510 LET tlt=ps-px: LET yc=y-1
9520 IF tlt<=0 THEN LET tlt=0: LET y=0: LET yc=0
9530 GO TO 9930
9540 PRINT "Enter BCOR.      BCOD.": INPUT r1,y1: P
RINT "         ";r1;" mm.",y1;" m
m.": LET r1=r1*20: LET y1=y1*10
9560 PRINT "Enter BPOR1.     BPOD1.": INPUT r2,y2:
PRINT "         ";r2;" mm.",y2;"
mm.": LET r2=r2*20: LET y2=y2*10
9580 PRINT "Enter BPOR2.     BPOD2.": INPUT r3,y3:
PRINT "         ";r3;" mm.",y3;"
mm.": LET r3=r3*20: LET y3=y3*10
9600 PRINT "Enter BPOR3.     BPOD3.": INPUT r4,y4:
PRINT "         ";r4;" mm.",y4;"
mm.": LET r4=r4*20: LET y4=y4*10
9620 PRINT : PRINT "Enter diameter for edge": PRIN
T "clearance.": INPUT yt: PRIN
T yt;" mm.": LET yt=yt*10
9630 RETURN
9700 REM aspheric
9710 PRINT "ASPHERIC LENS."
9720 PRINT : PRINT "Enter lens vertex radius.": IN
PUT r1: PRINT r1;" mm.": LET r
1=r1*20
9730 PRINT "Enter axial edge lift.": INPUT z: PRIN
T z;" mm.": LET z=z*20
9740 PRINT "Enter diameter for edge lift.": INPUT
yt: PRINT yt;" mm.": LET yt=yt
*10
9745 REM lens equations
9750 LET x1=r1-SQR (r1*r1-yt*yt)-z
9760 LET p1=((2*r1*x1)-(yt*yt))/(x1*x1)
9770 LET rs=r1/p1
```

198 Computer programs

```
9775 REM corneal equation
9780 LET rr=ro/p
9785 LET xct=rr-SQR (rr*rr-(yt*yt)/p)
9790 REM loop for sags
9795 REM contact lens
9800 LET pxc=0: LET px2=0
9805 CLS : PRINT "COMPUTING NOW."
9810 FOR y=1 TO yt
9820 LET x2=rs-SQR (rs*rs-(y*y)/p1)
9830 LET dif=x2-px2
9840 LET px2=x2
9845 REM cornea
9850 LET xc=rr-SQR (rr*rr-(y*y)/p)
9860 LET difc=xc-pxc
9870 LET pxc=xc
9880 IF difc>=(dif+.0001) THEN LET tlt=px2-pxc: LE
T yc=y-2: GO TO 9920
9890 BEEP .01,50
9900 NEXT y
9910 LET tlt=px2-pxc: LET yc=y-1
9920 IF tlt<=0 THEN LET tlt=0: LET y=0: LET yc=0
9930 LET xct=xct/20: LET x1=x1/20
9940 LET tlt=tlt/20: LET tlt=INT (tlt*1000+.5)/100
0
9950 LET e=xct+tlt-x1: LET e=INT (e*1000+.5)/1000:
 LET xct=INT (xct*1000+.5)/100
0
9960 PRINT : PRINT "TLT = ";tlt;" mm.": PRINT : PR
INT "CONTACT DIAMETER = ";yc/1
0;" mm.": PRINT
9970 PRINT "AXIAL EDGE CLEARANCE = ";e;" mm."
9980 PRINT "at diameter ";yt/10;" mm."
9985 PRINT : PRINT "Prim. sag of cornea = ";xct;"
mm."
9990 GO TO 8950
```

In order to check the program try the following:

(1) Enter corneal radius   enter 7.4
    Enter p value for cornea   enter .8
    Is the lens an aspheric? y/n   enter n
    Is the lens an offset bicurve? y/n   enter n
    Enter BCOR   enter 7.6
          BCOD   enter 6.5
    Enter BPOR.1   enter 10.5
          BPOD.1   enter 8.5
    Enter BPOR.2   enter Ø
          BPOD.2   enter Ø

Enter BPOR.3	enter 0
BPOD.3	enter 0
Enter diameter for edge clearance	enter 8.5
This should result in:	
TLT	0 mm
Contact diameter	0 mm
Axial edge clearance at diameter 8.5 mm	0.201 mm
Primary sag of cornea	1.314 mm

(2)
Enter corneal radius	enter 7.6
Enter p value for cornea	enter 0.8
Is the lens an aspheric? y/n	enter n
Is the lens an offset bicurve? y/n	enter n
Enter BCOR	enter 7.8
BCOD	enter 7
Enter BPOR.1	enter 8.8
BPOD.1	enter 8
Enter BPOR.2	enter 11
BPOD.2	enter 8.6
Enter BPOR.3	enter 0
BPOD.3	enter 0
Enter diameter for edge clearance	enter 8.6
This should result in:	
TLT	0 mm
Contact diameter	0 mm
Axial edge clearance at diameter 8.60 mm	0.119 mm
Primary sag of cornea	1.306 mm

(3)
Enter corneal radius	enter 8
Enter p value for cornea	enter .8
Is the lens aspheric? y/n	enter n
Is the lens an offset bicurve? y/n	enter n
Enter BCOR	enter 7.8
BCOD	enter 7
Enter BPOR.1	enter 8.8
BPOD.1	enter 8
Enter BPOR.2	enter 11
BPOD.2	enter 8.6
Enter BPOR.3	enter 12.25
BPOD.3	enter 9

Enter diameter for edge clearance	enter 9
This should result in:	
TLT	0.032 mm
Contact diameter	7 mm
Axial edge clearance at diameter 9 mm	0.126 mm
Primary sag of cornea	1.358 mm

(4)
Enter corneal radius	enter 7.4
Enter p value	enter .8
Is the lens an aspheric? y/n	enter n
Is the lens an offset bicurve? y/n	enter y
Enter BCOR	enter 7.35
BCOD	enter 6.5
Enter axial edge lift	enter .1
Enter diameter for edge lift	enter 9.25

The computer will now calculate the BPORs that produce the requested axial edge lift. This may take some time.

Select a suitable BPOR	enter 13.65
This should result in:	
TLT	0.016 mm
Contact diameter	6.9 mm
Axial edge clearance	0.059 mm
Primary sag of cornea	1.58 mm

(5)
Enter corneal radius	enter 8
Enter p value for cornea	enter .8
Is the lens an aspheric? y/n	enter y
Enter lens vertex radius	enter 7.8
Enter axial edge lift	enter .12
Enter diameter for edge lift	enter 9
This should result in:	
TLT	0.004 mm
Contact diameter	4.2 mm
Axial edge clearance at diameter 9 mm	0.053 mm
Primary sag of cornea	1.358 mm

7.10 Lenticular edge thickness (lines 1500–1990)

This program calculates the axial thickness at the junction of a lenticulated lens and then indicates the axial edge thickness for any front peripheral radius that the user selects. The assumption is made that the junction diameter, i.e. the front central optic diameter FCOD, is equal to the BCOD. The program will handle C2, C3 and C4 lenses.

The user is asked to enter the number of back surface curves. This is followed by a request for the BVP; the centre thickness; the refractive index; and finally the back surface specification given in the usual way, working through radius and diameter from the lens centre to the periphery. The computer then displays the front surface radius and the junction thickness to three decimal places. This is followed by an option to repeat the exercise which allows the user to enter an alternative centre thickness, e.g. where the junction thickness is too large or too small. If this option is rejected the computer asks for the front peripheral optic radius FPOR and, when this is entered, it displays the axial edge thickness to three decimal places. The computer then asks if the user wishes to try an alternative FPOR in order to alter the axial edge thickness to a more acceptable value, should this be necessary. The final option is to repeat the whole exercise for another lens.

The full listing of the program is given below.

```
1500 REM lentic
1505 DIM r(10): DIM d(10)
1510 CLS
1520 PRINT : PRINT "LENTICULAR EDGE THICKNESS."
1530 PRINT : PRINT "This section computes the"
1540 PRINT "design of a lenticular carrier"
1550 PRINT "zone.It assumes that FCOD=BCOD."
1560 PRINT : PRINT "How many back surface curves?"
1570 INPUT c: PRINT "C";c
1580 IF c<2 THEN PRINT "NOT AVAILABLE": GO TO 1570
1590 IF c>4 THEN PRINT "NOT AVAILABLE": GO TO 1570
1600 PRINT : PRINT "enter lens specification:"
1610 PRINT : PRINT "enter BVP ": INPUT f: PRINT f;
" D."
1620 PRINT "enter required centre thickness": INPU
T tc: PRINT tc;" mm."
1630 PRINT "enter lens refractive index": INPUT n:
 PRINT n
1640 PRINT : PRINT "BCOR               BCOD": INPUT r
(1),d(1): PRINT r(1),d(1)
1650 FOR i=2 TO c
1660 PRINT "BPOR";i-1;"            BPOD";i-1: INPUT
 r(i),d(i): PRINT r(i),d(i)
1670 NEXT i
1680 REM compute front surface radius
1690 LET f1=(1-n)*1000/r(1)
```

Computer programs

```
1700 LET l=1000/((1000/(f-f1))+(tc/n))
1710 LET rf=(n-1)*1000/l
1720 LET rf=INT (rf*100+.5)/100
1730 REM compute junction thickness
1740 LET sf=rf-SQR (rf*rf-(d(1)/2)*(d(1)/2))
1750 LET so=r(1)-SQR (r(1)*r(1)-(d(1)/2)*(d(1)/2))
1760 LET tj=INT ((tc+so-sf)*1000+.5)/1000
1770 PRINT : PRINT "Front surface radius is",rf;" mm."
1780 PRINT "Junction axial thickness is",tj;" mm."
1790 PRINT : PRINT "Another specification?(y/n)": INPUT q$
1800 IF q$="y" THEN GO TO 1600
1810 IF q$="Y" THEN GO TO 1600
1820 REM compute sags and edge thickness
1830 LET p=0
1840 FOR i=2 TO c
1850 LET s1=r(i)-SQR (r(i)*r(i)-(d(i)/2)*(d(i)/2))
1860 LET s2=r(i)-SQR (r(i)*r(i)-(d(i-1)/2)*(d(i-1)/2))
1870 LET p=p+s1-s2
1880 NEXT i
1890 LET p=p+so
1900 PRINT : PRINT "enter the FPOR": INPUT rp: PRINT rp;" mm."
1910 LET s3=rp-SQR (rp*rp-(d(c)/2)*(d(c)/2))
1920 LET s4=rp-SQR (rp*rp-(d(1)/2)*(d(1)/2))
1930 LET te=p-so-s3+s4+tj
1940 LET te=INT (te*1000+.5)/1000
1950 PRINT : PRINT "The axial edge thickness is",te;" mm."
1960 PRINT : PRINT "another FPOR?(y/n)": INPUT q$
1965 IF q$="y" THEN GO TO 1900
1970 IF q$="Y" THEN GO TO 1900
1975 PRINT : PRINT "another lens?(y/n)": INPUT q$
1980 IF q$="y" THEN GO TO 1510
1985 IF q$="Y" THEN GO TO 1510
1990 RETURN
```

In order to check the program try the following:

How many back surface curves	enter 2
BVP	enter 13
Required centre thickness	enter .3
Refractive index	enter 1.49
BCOR	enter 7.8
BCOD	enter 6.5
BPOR.1	enter 8.3
BPOD.1	enter 9

This should result in:

Front surface radius	6.56 mm
Junction thickness	0.148 mm
Another specification	enter n
FPOR	enter 10

The edge thickness should be 0.284 mm.

7.11 The RC device (lines 2500–2660)

This program converts the focimeter reading immediately into a BCOR for the lens under investigation.

The user is asked to enter the convex surface radius of the RC device followed by its central thickness. This means that the program will work for any RC device that a practitioner cares to have made. The computer then asks for the contact lens central thickness followed by the FVP of the system which will be the focimeter reading, at the end point. The computer then prints the BCOR of the contact lens to two decimal places.

The full program listing is given below.

```
2500 REM R-C
2510 CLS
2520 PRINT : PRINT "THE R-C DEVICE."
2530 PRINT : PRINT "enter convex surface radius of
"
2540 PRINT "the R-C device": INPUT r1: PRINT r1;"
mm."
2550 PRINT "enter thickness of ": PRINT "the R-C d
evice": INPUT t1: PRINT t1;" m
m."
2560 PRINT : PRINT "enter the lens central": PRINT
" thickness": INPUT t2: PRINT
t2;" mm."
2570 PRINT "enter FVP indicated by": PRINT "focime
ter": INPUT fv: PRINT fv;" D."
2580 LET l2=1000/((490/r1)-fv)
2590 LET t=(t1+t2)/1.49
2600 LET f2=-1000/(l2-t)
2610 LET r2=INT ((-490/f2)*100+.5)/100
2620 PRINT : PRINT "The BCOR is ",r2;" mm."
2630 PRINT : PRINT "repeat?(y/n)": INPUT q$
2640 IF q$="y" THEN GO TO 2560
2650 IF q$="Y" THEN GO TO 2560
2660 RETURN
```

In order to check the program try the following:

Radius of RC device	enter 8
RC device thickness	enter .5
Lens central thickness	enter .1
FVP indicated by focimeter	enter 6

This should give a BCOR of 8.67 mm.

N.B. The RC device can only be used on **PMMA** lenses where the refractive index is 1.490. However, some alterations to the above program could extend its use to contact lenses of any refractive index.

7.12 The menu (lines 10–390)

This menu is designed to be merged with all the other programs described so far in this chapter and this provides the practitioner with a single program which lists ten options in the menu. At the end of any option the user is returned to the menu. All the merged programs use approximately 20K of the computer's memory. Line 20 is a command peculiar to the Sinclair Spectrum which instructs the computer to produce a sound every time that a key is pressed. This is a useful facility, when entering data, which helps to ensure that the user always depresses the computer keys fully.

The full program listing is given below.

```
  5 REM c12

 10 REM OPTICS OF CONTACT
 15 REM LENSES by Bill Douthwaite
 16 REM and Jim Gilchrist.
 20 CLEAR : POKE 23609,35
 90 DIM r(10): DIM d(10): DIM o(10): DIM z(10)
110 PRINT "CONTACT LENS OPTICS."
120 PRINT "by Douthwaite and Gilchrist."
130 PRINT : PRINT "Tests available :-"
140 PRINT "1.  Lens effective power."
150 PRINT "2.  r/F in air conversion."
160 PRINT "3.  r/F interface conversion."
170 PRINT "4.  F.V.P. and r1."
180 PRINT "5.  Peripheral radii for"
185 PRINT "    specific   edge lift."
190 PRINT "6.  Edge thickness and lift in a"
195 PRINT "    given lens."
200 PRINT "7.  Periph radius for offset of"
205 PRINT "    given edge lift."
```

```
210 PRINT "8.  Calculate x and p for"
215 PRINT "      aspheric surface."
220 PRINT "9.  Calculate TLT and axial edge"
225 PRINT "      clearance."
230 PRINT "10. Edge thickness in a"
235 PRINT "      lenticular."
240 PRINT "11. The R-C device."
250 PRINT : INPUT "which test?";ee
260 IF ee<1 THEN PRINT "NOT AVAILABLE": PAUSE 100: CLS : GO TO 110
265 IF ee>11 THEN PRINT "NOT AVAILABLE": PAUSE 100: CLS : GO TO 110
270 IF ee=1 THEN GO SUB 1000
280 IF ee=2 THEN GO SUB 2000
290 IF ee=3 THEN GO SUB 3000
300 IF ee=4 THEN GO SUB 4000
310 IF ee=5 THEN GO SUB 5000
320 IF ee=6 THEN GO SUB 6000
330 IF ee=7 THEN GO SUB 7000
340 IF ee=8 THEN GO SUB 8000
350 IF ee=9 THEN GO SUB 9000
360 IF ee=10 THEN GO SUB 1500
370 IF ee=11 THEN GO SUB 2500
380 GO TO 20
390 STOP
```

7.13 Lens thickness

This program cannot be merged with the others. It allows calculation of lens thickness and can be applied to hard, GPH and soft contact lenses with monocurve, bicurve, tricurve, four curve, offset or aspheric back surfaces. The program calculates radial thickness (radial to the front surface of the lens) and displays a radial thickness profile of the lens during the time that the program is running (this includes markers for the transition positions), and when this has been completed the following thicknesses are specified to three decimal places:

(1) radial edge thickness;
(2) maximum radial thickness;
(3) arithmetic mean radial thickness;
(4) harmonic mean radial thickness.

  (1) is self-explanatory. (2) is the maximum radial thickness encountered during the calculations. (3) is a useful value for giving the practitioner some idea of the physical dimensions of the lens which is more realistic than a centre or edge thickness. (4) is the

value required when considering the gas flow through the lens, since this is proportional to $1/t$ where t is the thickness. If we take the average of the $1/t$ values acquired and then take the reciprocal of this mean, we have the harmonic mean thickness. The program calculates the radial thickness from the centre of the lens to the edge at points which are spaced at 0.05 mm intervals across the semi-diameter of the lens. In the case of the offset lens the computer must search for a suitable BPOR using a subroutine based on the program described in Section 7.7. This section runs from line 900 to line 1100. In the case of the aspheric back surface curves, the program can only deal with ellipsoids and paraboloids (i.e. where p has a positive value). If the practitioner wishes to examine a monocurve design then he or she should request the C2 lens option and enter the same value for the BCOR and BPOR. In these circumstances the BCOD value entered will have no bearing on the calculations.

There is also a section in this program which concerns the need to lenticulate negative lenses. If the BVP is negative the computer asks what is the maximum thickness that the practitioner is prepared to accept. When the value has been entered the computer will display the diameter at which this thickness first occurs. The practitioner may then use this as the FCOD for lenticulation purposes, or consider an alternative central thickness.

The full program listing is given below.

```
   5 REM mean t
  10 CLS
  15 CLEAR : POKE 23609,35
  18 DIM r(10): DIM d(10)
  20 LET t1=10
  40 PRINT : PRINT "RADIAL LENS THICKNESS.": PRINT
"by Bill Douthwaite": PRINT "
and Jim Gilchrist"
  50 PRINT : PRINT "enter lens BVP ": INPUT f: PRI
NT f;" D."
  60 IF f>=0 THEN GO TO 130
 110 PRINT : PRINT "enter maximum acceptable": PRI
NT "thickness before lenticula
ting"
 120 INPUT t1: PRINT t1;" mm."
 130 PRINT : PRINT "enter refractive index ": INPU
T n: PRINT n
 135 CLS : PRINT : PRINT "select lens type :"
 140 PRINT : PRINT "1. C2"
 150 PRINT "2. C3"
 160 PRINT "3. C4"
 170 PRINT "4. CONTRALATERAL OFFSET BICURVE"
```

Lens thickness

```
 180 PRINT "5. ASPHERIC"
 190 PRINT "option?": INPUT t
 200 IF t<1 THEN PRINT "NOT AVAILABLE": GO TO 190
 210 IF t>5 THEN PRINT "NOT AVAILABLE": GO TO 190
 220 IF t<4 THEN GO SUB 400
 230 IF t=4 THEN GO SUB 900
 240 IF t=5 THEN GO SUB 1500
 250 PRINT : PRINT "Another lens?(y/n)": INPUT q$
 260 IF q$="y" THEN GO TO 10
 270 IF q$="Y" THEN GO TO 10
 280 STOP
 300 REM radial edge result
 305 LET tt=INT ((tt/za)*1000+.5)/1000
 310 LET th=INT ((za/th)*1000+.5)/1000
 320 LET tr=INT (tr*1000+.5)/1000
 330 LET tm=INT (tm*1000+.5)/1000
 340 PRINT : PRINT "RADIAL THICKNESS (mm) :"
 350 PRINT "edge= ";tr;" max= ";tm
 370 PRINT "arith.mean= ";tt: PRINT "harm.mean= ";th
 390 RETURN
 400 REM C2 C3 AND C4 ROUTINES
 410 CLS
 420 PRINT : PRINT "C2, C3 AND C4 LENSES."
 430 PRINT : PRINT "enter the lens specification:"
 440 PRINT "BCOR              BCOD": INPUT r(1),d(1): PRINT r(1),d(1)
 450 FOR i=2 TO t+1
 460 PRINT "BPOR";i-1;"           BPOD";i-1: INPUT r(i),d(i): PRINT r(i),d(i)
 470 NEXT i
 480 PRINT "enter centre thickness ": INPUT tc: PRINT tc;" mm."
 485 LET tt=0: LET th=0: LET za=0: LET tm=0: LET te=0: LET tr=0: LET tj=0
 490 CLS
 500 LET f2=(1-n)*1000/r(1)
 510 LET 12=1000/((1000/(f-f2))+(tc/n))
 520 LET rf=(n-1)*1000/12
 530 REM compute radial parameters
 535 LET s2=0: LET s3=0: LET s4=0
 536 LET s5=0: LET s6=0: LET s7=0
 540 FOR i=1 TO t+1
 550 IF i=1 THEN LET ba=1
 560 IF i>1 THEN LET ba=d(i-1)*10
 570 FOR j=ba TO 500
 580 LET y=j/20: LET za=za+1: LET tt=tt+tr
 590 IF i=1 THEN LET yy=y
 595 IF i>1 THEN LET yy=d(1)/2
 600 LET s1=r(1)-SQR (r(1)*r(1)-yy*yy)
```

```
610 LET sf=rf-SQR (rf*rf-y*y)
620 IF i=1 THEN GO TO 730
630 IF i<4 THEN GO TO 660
640 LET s6=r(4)-SQR (r(4)*r(4)-y*y)
650 LET s7=r(4)-SQR (r(4)*r(4)-(d(3)/2*d(3)/2))
660 IF i<3 THEN GO TO 700
670 IF i=3 THEN LET yy=y
675 IF i>3 THEN LET yy=d(3)/2
680 LET s4=r(3)-SQR (r(3)*r(3)-yy*yy)
690 LET s5=r(3)-SQR (r(3)*r(3)-(d(2)/2)*(d(2)/2))
700 IF i=2 THEN LET yy=y
705 IF i>2 THEN LET yy=d(2)/2
710 LET s2=r(2)-SQR (r(2)*r(2)-yy*yy)
720 LET s3=r(2)-SQR (r(2)*r(2)-(d(1)/2)*(d(1)/2))
730 LET ts=s1+s2-s3+s4-s5+s6-s7
740 LET tj=ts+tc-sf
750 LET rv=ATN (y/(rf-tj-sf))
760 LET tr=rf-(y/SIN (rv))
770 LET th=th+1/tr
775 IF tr<=0 THEN PRINT "LENS TOO THIN": GO TO 480
780 IF tr>tm THEN LET tm=tr
790 IF tr>=tl THEN PRINT tl;" mm thick at diam. ";2*y;" mm."
795 IF tr>=tl THEN LET tl=10
800 IF y>=(d(i)/2) THEN GO TO 815
805 LET tg=tr*300: LET gr=y*20: PLOT gr,0: DRAW 0,tg
810 NEXT j
815 PLOT gr-.5,0: INVERSE 1: DRAW 0,10: INVERSE 0
820 NEXT i
825 GO SUB 300
830 PRINT : PRINT "another thickness?(y/n)": INPUT q$
840 IF q$="y" AND f<0 THEN INPUT "max.thick.before lenticulating",tl: GO TO 480
845 IF q$="y" THEN GO TO 480
850 IF q$="Y" AND f<0 THEN INPUT "max.thickness before lenticulating";tl: GO TO 480
855 IF q$="Y" THEN GO TO 480
860 RETURN
900 REM offset lens routine
905 CLS
910 PRINT : PRINT "OFFSET BICURVE LENS."
915 PRINT : PRINT "enter axial edge lift": INPUT z
920 LET z=INT (z*1000+.5)/1000
925 PRINT : PRINT "enter BCOR": INPUT r(1): PRINT r(1);" mm."
```

```
 930 PRINT : PRINT "enter BCOD": INPUT d(1): PRINT
d(1);" mm."
 935 PRINT : PRINT "enter diameter for edge lift":
INPUT d(2): PRINT d(2);" mm."
 940 CLS : PRINT "COMPUTING THE BPOR"
 945 FOR i=r(1)*140 TO 6000 STEP 5
 948 BEEP .05,55
 950 LET r2=i/100
 955 LET s1=r(1)-SQR (r(1)*r(1)-(d(1)/2)*(d(1)/2))
 960 LET s2=r(1)-SQR (r(1)*r(1)-(d(2)/2)*(d(2)/2))
 965 LET yy=(d(1)/2)/r(1)*(r2-r(1))
 970 LET y2=d(1)/2+yy: LET y3=d(2)/2+yy
 975 LET s3=r2-SQR (r2*r2-y2*y2)
 980 LET s4=r2-SQR (r2*r2-y3*y3)
 985 LET e=(s2-s1)-(s4-s3): LET e=INT (e*1000+.5)/
1000
 990 IF e=z THEN PRINT r2
 995 IF e>z THEN GO TO 1105
1100 NEXT i
1105 PRINT "These are the BPORs for the": PRINT "r
equired edge lift."
1110 PRINT : PRINT "Select a suitable BPOR": INPUT
 r(2)
1120 PRINT : PRINT "enter centre thickness": INPUT
 tc
1122 CLS : PRINT "OFFSET BICURVE."
1123 LET tt=0: LET th=0: LET za=0: LET tm=0: LET t
e=0: LET tr=0: LET tj=0
1125 LET f2=(1-n)*1000/r(1)
1130 LET l2=1000/((1000/(f-f2))+(tc/n))
1135 LET rf=(n-1)*1000/l2
1140 LET of=(((d(1)/2)/r(1))*r(2))-(d(1)/2)
1145 LET s2=0: LET s3=0
1150 FOR i=1 TO 2
1160 IF i=1 THEN LET ba=1
1170 IF i>1 THEN LET ba=d(1)*10
1180 FOR j=ba TO 500
1190 LET y=j/20: LET za=za+1: LET tt=tt+tr
1195 LET y2=y+of: LET y3=(d(1)/2)+of
1200 IF i=1 THEN LET yy=y
1210 IF i>1 THEN LET yy=d(1)/2
1220 LET s1=r(1)-SQR (r(1)*r(1)-yy*yy)
1230 LET sf=rf-SQR (rf*rf-y*y)
1235 IF i=1 THEN GO TO 1260
1240 LET s2=r(2)-SQR (r(2)*r(2)-y2*y2)
1250 LET s3=r(2)-SQR (r(2)*r(2)-y3*y3)
1260 LET ts=s1+s2-s3
1270 LET tj=ts+tc-sf
1280 LET rv=ATN (y/(rf-tj-sf))
1290 LET tr=rf-(y/SIN (rv))
```

210 Computer programs

```
1300 LET th=th+1/tr
1310 IF tr<=0 THEN PRINT : PRINT "LENS TOO THIN":
GO TO 1120
1320 IF tr>tm THEN LET tm=tr
1330 IF tr>=tl THEN PRINT tl;" mm thick at diam. "
;2*y;" mm."
1340 IF tr>=tl THEN LET tl=10
1350 IF y>=(d(i)/2) THEN GO TO 1365
1355 LET tg=tr*300: LET gr=y*20: PLOT gr,0: DRAW 0
,tg
1360 NEXT j
1365 PLOT gr-.5,0: INVERSE 1: DRAW 0,10: INVERSE 0
1370 NEXT i
1380 GO SUB 300: REM results
1390 PRINT : PRINT "another thickness?(y/n)": INPU
T q$
1395 IF q$="y" AND f<0 THEN INPUT "max.thick.for l
enticulation",tl: GO TO 1120
1400 IF q$="y" THEN GO TO 1120
1405 IF q$="Y" AND f<0 THEN INPUT "max.thick.for l
enticulation",tl: GO TO 1120
1410 IF q$="Y" THEN GO TO 1120
1420 RETURN
1500 REM ASPHERIC LENS ROUTINE
1510 CLS
1520 PRINT : PRINT "ASPHERIC LENS."
1525 PRINT : PRINT "enter vertex radius": INPUT r1
: PRINT r1;" mm."
1530 PRINT : PRINT "enter axial edge lift": INPUT
z: PRINT z;" mm."
1535 PRINT : PRINT "enter diameter for edge lift":
 INPUT d1: PRINT d1;" mm."
1540 LET s=r1-SQR (r1*r1-(d1/2)*(d1/2))
1545 LET x=s-z
1550 LET p=(2*x*r1)-((d1/2)*(d1/2))
1555 LET p=p/(x*x)
1560 PRINT : PRINT "enter centre thickness": INPUT
 tc: PRINT tc;" mm."
1563 CLS : PRINT "ASPHERIC LENS."
1564 LET tt=0: LET th=0: LET za=0: LET tm=0: LET t
e=0: LET tr=0: LET tj=0
1565 LET f2=(1-n)*1000/r1
1570 LET l2=1000/((1000/(f-f2))+(tc/n))
1575 LET rf=(n-1)*1000/l2
1580 FOR i=1 TO 900
1585 LET y=i/20: LET za=za+1: LET tt=tt+tr
1590 LET sf=rf-SQR (rf*rf-y*y)
1595 LET ps=r1/p-SQR ((r1/p)*(r1/p)-(y*y)/p)
1600 LET tj=ps+tc-sf: LET rv=ATN (y/(rf-tj-sf))
1605 LET tr=rf-(y/SIN (rv))
```

```
1610 LET th=th+1/tr
1612 IF tr<=0 THEN PRINT : PRINT "LENS TOO THIN":
GO TO 1560
1615 IF tr>tm THEN LET tm=tr
1620 IF tr>=tl THEN PRINT tl;" mm thick at diam. "
;2*y;" mm."
1625 IF tr>=tl THEN LET tl=10
1630 IF y>=(d1/2) THEN GO TO 1640
1632 LET tg=tr*300: LET gr=y*20: PLOT gr,0: DRAW 0
,tg
1635 NEXT i
1640 GO SUB 300: REM results
1645 PRINT : PRINT "another thickness?(y/n)": INPU
T q$
1648 IF q$="y" AND f<0 THEN INPUT "max.thick.for l
enticulation",tl: GO TO 1560
1650 IF q$="y" THEN GO TO 1560
1655 IF q$="Y" AND f<0 THEN INPUT "max.thick.for l
enticulation",tl: GO TO 1560
1660 IF q$="Y" THEN GO TO 1560
1670 RETURN
```

The PLOT and DRAW commands in the above program are specifically for the Sinclair Spectrum. These lines instruct the computer to draw a series of vertical lines which run from the left of the screen to the right, with the length of each line indicating the contact lens radial thickness at a given eccentricity. This results in the computer drawing a radial thickness profile which starts at the centre of the contact lens (on the left side of the screen) and describes the radial thickness changes as the calculations proceed towards the lens periphery. The lines which also contain the command INVERSE mark the position of the lens transitions by removing a short section of the line drawn for that particular region of the contact lens. The practitioner will need to familiarize himself or herself with the computer's graphics where a machine other than the Spectrum is used and modify these lines accordingly.

In order to check the program try the following:

(1) BVP   enter −6.37
    Maximum acceptable thickness   enter   .25
    Refractive index   enter 1.49
    Lens type   enter 1
    BCOR   enter 7.6
    BCOD   enter 6.5
    BPOR.1   enter 10.5
    BPOD.1   enter 8.5
    Centre thickness   enter .2

The computer will then display the lens profile and mark the transition. It should state that the 0.25 mm thickness occurs at a diameter of 5.9 mm. When the profile is complete is should display:

Edge thickness	0.15 mm
Maximum thickness	0.262 mm
Arithmetic mean thickness	0.216 mm
Harmonic mean thickness	0.215 mm

If the alternative thickness option now offered is accepted, then when the new centre thickness is entered the computer will repeat the exercise without the need to re-enter the parameters apart from the maximum acceptable thickness for lenticulation.

(2)
BVP	enter −	4.75
Maximum acceptable thickness	enter	.23
Refractive index	enter	1.49
Lens type	enter	2
BCOR	enter	7.8
BCOD	enter	7
BPOR.1	enter	8.8
BPOD.1	enter	8
BPOR.2	enter	11
BPOD.2	enter	8.6
Centre thickness	enter	.2

The computer should state that the 0.23 mm thickness occurs at diameter 5.5 mm and give the following:

Edge thickness	0.189 mm
Maximum thickness	0.25 mm
Arithmetic mean thickness	0.217 mm
Harmonic mean thickness	0.218 mm

(3)
BVP	enter	2
Refractive index	enter	1.49
Lens type	enter	3
BCOR	enter	7.8
BCOD	enter	7
BPOR.1	enter	8.8
BPOD.1	enter	8
BPOR.2	enter	11
BPOD.2	enter	8.6
BPOR.3	enter	12.25
BPOD.3	enter	9.5
Centre thickness	enter	.3

The computer should display the following:
Edge thickness   0.012 mm
Maximum thickness   0.3 mm
Arithmetic mean thickness   0.248 mm
Harmonic mean thickness   0.173 mm

(4) BVP   enter −4
    Maximum acceptable thickness   enter   .23
    Refractive index   enter   1.49
    Lens type   enter   4
    Axial edge lift   enter   .12
    BCOR   enter   7.2
    BCOD   enter   6.5
    Diameter for edge lift   enter   9.5
    The computer will now calculate suitable BPORs.
    Select BPOR   enter   12.65
    Centre thickness   enter   .2
    The computer should state that the thickness of 0.23 mm occurs at diameter 6.3 mm and also:
    Edge thickness   0.183 mm
    Maximum thickness   0.236 mm
    Arithmetic mean thickness   0.212 mm
    Harmonic mean thickness   0.213 mm

(5) BVP   enter −4
    Maximum acceptable thickness   enter   .21
    Refractive index   enter   1.49
    Lens type   enter   5
    Vertex radius   enter   7.2
    Axial edge lift   enter   .12
    Diameter for edge lift   enter   9.5
    Centre thickness   enter   .2
    The computer should state that the thickness of 0.21 mm occurs at diameter 4.3 mm and also:
    Edge thickness   0.183 mm
    Maximum thickness   0.214 mm
    Arithmetic mean thickness   0.204 mm
    Harmonic mean thickness   0.206 mm

The programs listed in this chapter have not received exhaustive use and may well possess bugs that the writer has not discovered. I would therefore be grateful to receive any comments or criticisms from contact lens practitioners.

References

ATKINSON, T. C. O. (1984). A reappraisal of the concept of fitting rigid hard lenses by the tear layer thickness and edge clearance technique. *J. Br. Cont. Lens Ass.* **7** (3), 106–110

BARON, H. (1975). Some remarks on the correction of astigmatic eyes by means of soft contact lenses. *Contacto* **19** (6), 4–8

BENNETT, A. G. (1966). The calibration of keratometers. *Optician* **151**, 317–322

BENNETT, A. G. (1968). Aspherical contact lens surfaces. *Ophthal. Optician* **8**, 1037–1040

BENNETT, A. G. (1976). Power changes of soft contact lenses due to bending. *Ophthal. Optician* **16**, 939–945

BENNETT, A. G. (1985). Relationship between front and back surfaces for a thick lens. In *Optics of Contact Lenses*, 5th Ed. pp. 27–29. London: Association of Dispensing Opticians

BENNETT, Q. (1965). Underwater contact lenses. *J. Br. Sub Aqua Club* (June), 26–27

DOUTHWAITE, W. A. (1971). Bifocal underwater contact lenses. *Ophthal. Optician* **11**, 10–14

EMSLEY, H. H. (1963). The keratometer: measurement of concave surfaces. *Optician* **146**, 161–168

GUILLON, M., LYDON, D. P. M. and SAMMONS, W. A. (1983). Designing rigid gas permeable contact lenses using the edge clearance technique. *J. Br. Cont. Lens Ass.* **6**(1), 19–26

GUILLON, M., CROSBIE-WALSH, J. and BYRNES, D. (1986). Application of pachometry to the measurement of hard contact lens edge profile. *Trans. Br. Cont. Lens Ass. Annu. Clin. Conf.*, 56–59

HODD, F. A. B. (1966). A design study of the back surface of corneal contact lenses. *Ophthal. Optician* **6**, 1175–1238; **7**, 14–39

MANDELL, R. B. (1974). Can gel lens power be measured accurately? *Internat. Contact Lens Clin.* **1**, 36–37

PEARSON, R. M. (1980). Measurement of centre thickness of soft lenses. *Ophthal. Optician* **20**, 778–782

PEARSON, R. M. (1986). How thick is a contact lens? *Trans. Br. Cont. Lens Ass. Annu. Clin. Conf.*, 82–86

RABBETTS, R. B. (1976). Large corneal lenses with constant axial edge lift. *Ophthal. Optician* **16**, 236–239

RUBEN, M. (1966). Use of conoidal curves in corneal contact lenses. *Br. J. Ophthal.* **50**, 642–645

SAMMONS, W. A. (1981). Thin lens design and average thickness. *J. Br. Cont. Lens Ass.* **4**(3), 90–97

SARVER, M. D. and KERR, K. (1964). A radius of curvature measuring device for contact lenses. *Am. J. Optom.* **41**, 481–489

STONE, J. (1975). Corneal lenses with constant axial edge lift. *Ophthal. Optician* **15**, 818–824

STONE, J. and FRANCIS, J. L. (1980). Practical optics of contact lenses and aspects of contact lens design. In *Contact Lenses*, ed. by J. Stone and J. L. Phillips, p. 114. London: Butterworths

STONE, J. and PHILLIPS, J. L. (1980). *Contact Lenses*. London: Butterworths

STRACHAN, J. P. F. (1973). Some principles of the optics of hydrophilic lenses and geometrical optics applied to flexible lenses. *Aus. J. Optom.* **56**, 25–33

TOMLINSON, A. and BIBBY, M. (1977). Corneal clearance at the apex and edge of a hard contact lens. *Int. Cont. Lens Clin.* **4**(6), 50–56

TOWNSLEY, M. (1970). New knowledge of the corneal contour. *Contacto* **14**(3), 38–43

WICHTERLE, O. (1967). Changes of refracting power of a soft lens caused by its flattening. In *Corneal and Scleral Contact Lenses—Proc. Int. Congress*, ed. by L. J. Girard, paper number 29, pp. 247–256. St Louis: Mosby

WINN, B., ACKERLEY, R. G., BROWN, C. A., MURRAY, F. K., PRAIS, J. and ST JOHN, M. F. (1986). The superiority of contact lenses in the correction of all anisometropia. *Trans. Br. Cont. Lens Ass. Annu. Clin. Conf.*, 95–100

Index

Accommodation, 3
  ocular, 4
  spectacle, 3
  spectacles and contact lenses compared, 9
Accommodation/convergence relationship, 26
Air cell lens, *see* Underwater lenses
Anisometropia, 22
  axial, 23
  refractive, 22
Aphakic correction, 114
  near vision correction, 117
Aspheric surfaces, 55
  checking by optical spherometer, 142
  corneal topography, 87
  primary sag, 56
  Zag value, *see* Edge lift
Astigmatism,
  corneal, *see* cornea
  induced, 92
  lenticular, 90
  residual, 90
Axial edge lift, *see* Edge lift

Back surface solid bifocals, *see* Bifocal contact lenses
Back vertex power (BVP), 6
  flexure, 12
  modification induced power changes, 39
  over refraction with lens of inappropriate BCOR, 35
  radius to power change approximate rule, 37
  scleral impression lenses, 46
  thickness changes, 42
  toric PMMA and GPH lenses, 92
  toric soft lenses, 130
Basic retinal image size, 12
Bifocal contact lenses, 106
  addition power in air, 111
  back surface solids, 110
  front surface solids, 106
  fused, 112
  underwater bifocal lens, *see* Underwater lenses
Bitoric lenses, *see* Back surface toric lenses
Blur circles, 11

Centre thickness, *see* Thickness
Computer programs,
  aspheric surfaces, 192
  axial edge lift, 182
  BPOR for an offset lens, 190
  edge thickness and edge lift, 186
  effective power, 176
  front surface radius and FVP, 180
  interface radius/power conversion, 179
  lens thickness, 205
  lenticular edge thickness, 200
  menu, 202
  radius/power conversion in air, 177
  RC device, 203
  TLT and axial edge clearance, 193
Conic section equation, 56
Constant edge lift fitting sets, 61

Index 217

Continuous bicurve, *see* Offset bicurve
Convergence, 23
Cornea,
 astigmatism, 89, 133
 topography, 87
 toric TLT and axial clearance, 99

Drysdale's method, 140

Edge clearance from the cornea,
 axial, 87
 radial, 87
 on toric cornea, 99
Edge lift, 51
 axial, 51
 measurement by optical spherometer, *see* Optical spherometer
 radial, 54
 radial to axial ratio, 55
 Z value, 56
Edge thickness, *see* Thickness
Entrance pupil of the eye, 14
Equivalent focal length, 16

Far point of the eye, 2
Field of fixation, *see* Motor field of view
Flexure, *see* Soft lenses
Fluid lens, 28
Focimeter, 151
 radius checking, 156
 wet cell checking, 152
Front surface solid bifocals, *see* Bifocal contact lenses
Front vertex power (FVP), 42
Fused bifocals, *see* Bifocal contact lenses

Gas permeability, *see* Permeability
Gas transmission, 138

Heine's scale, 46

Induced astigmatism, *see* Astigmatism

Jack in the box effect, 116

Keratometer, 66
 checking concave surfaces, 80, 145
 doubling, 69
 equation, 67
 extending the range of measurement, 76, 146
 mire image formation, 71
 one and two position instruments, 75
 power scale, 78
 precautions, 81
 telecentric instrument, 72
 topographic instrument, 81
 wet cell checking of soft lenses, 147

Lens thickness, *see* Thickness
Lenticular astigmatism, *see* Astigmatism
Lenticular lenses, 117
Low vision aid telescope, 120
 magnification, *see* Magnification
 Motorfield of view, *see* Motor field of view
 near vision, 125
 telecon system, 124

Magnification, 12
 aphakic eyes, 116
 contact lens magnification, 14
 low vision aid telescope, 121
 refractive ametropia, 22
 relative spectacle magnification axial ametropia, 21
 spectacle magnification, 13
 total spectacle magnification, 19
Metre angle, 24
Modifying and existing lens, 39
 change in BVP due to change of thickness, *see* Back vertex power
 change in BVP due to damage of BCOR, *see* Back vertex power
Motor field of view, 114
 with LVA telescope, 122

Offset bicurve, 58
Optical spherometer,
   diameter measurement, 143
   edge lift measurement, 143
   radius measurement, 140
   thickness measurement, 142
   toric radii, *see* Toric surfaces
   wet cell measurement, 143
Orientation,
   contact lens, 98
   keratometer, *see* Keratometer
Over refraction, 29
   using inappropriate BCOR, *see* Back vertex power
Oxygen permeability, *see* Permeability
Oxygen transmission, *see* Gas transmission

Pachometer, 84
   doubling, 85
   precautions, 85
   thickness of a contact lens, 159
Permeability, 138
Photokeratoscope, 83
Power, 1
   effective power, 1
   see also Back vertex power
Primary optic diameter, *see* Scleral lenses
Primary sag of a contact lens, 51
Principal focus, 2
Principal planes, 15
Prism dioptre, 24
Prismatic effects, 61
   see also Convergence

Radial edge lift, *see* Edge lift
Radius checking device, *see* Focimeter
Radiuscope, *see* Optical spherometer
Radius of curvature, 29
   BCOR to BVP relationship, approximate rule for, *see* Back vertex power
   bifocal contact lenses,
     back surface, 110
     front surface, 106
   depression curve of fused bifocal, 112
   radius checking device, *see* Focimeter
   surface radii relationship in a thick lens, 31
   toric lenses, *see* Toric surfaces
Reduced thicknesses, *see* thickness
Residual astigmatism, *see* Astigmatism

Sag equation, 48
Scleral lenses,
   keratometer measurement of scleral radius, *see* Extending keratometer
   primary optic diameter, 160
   range of measurement, *see under* Keratometer
   tolerances, *see* Tolerances
Shape factor, 16
Soft lenses, 127
   astigmatism, 130
   corneal astigmatism, 133
   flexure equation, *see* Back vertex power
   power measurement by wet cell, *see* Focimeter
   radius measurement by wet cell, *see* Optical spherometer
   tolerances, *see* Tolerances
   toric lenses, *see* Toric surfaces
Spherometer, 149
'Step along' method, 17

Tear lens thickness, *see* Thickness
Telescope, *see* Low vision aid telescope
Thickness, 48
   axial tear lens, 87
   centre, 48
   edge, 48
   harmonic mean, 138
   mean, 138
   measurement by optical spherometer, *see* Optical spherometer

Thickness—*cont.*
  radial, 136
  reduced, 10
Tolerances,
  corneal lenses,
    BCOD, 166
    BCOR, 162
    bifocal add, 170
    BPOD, 166
    BPOR, 166
    BVP, 167
    central thickness, 168
    centration, 170
    cylinder axis, 168
    cylinder power, 168
    edge form, 169
    edge lift, 170
    edge thickness, 169
    FCOD, 170
    FCOR, 169
    FROR, 170
    OS, 167
    prism, 167
    segment height, 170
    toric surface radii, 168
  scleral lenses,
    back, scleral radius, 171
    BCOD, 171
    BCOR, 171
    BPOD, 171
    BPOR, 171
    BVP, 172
    central thickness, 172
    centration, 172
    clearance from cast, 172
    cylinder axis, 168
    cylinder power, 172
    FCOD, 172
    FCOR, 172
    OS, 171
    primary optic diameter, 171
    prism, 172
    toric surface radii, 172
  soft lenses,
    BCOD, 173
    BCOR, 172
    BPOD, 173
    BPOR, 173
    BVP, 173
    central thickness, 173
    centration, 174
    cylinder axis, 173
    cylinder power, 173
    edge thickness, 174
    FCOD, 174
    OS, 173
    prism, 173
Toric surfaces,
  back surface, hard, 91
  back surface, soft, 131
  checking by optical spherometer,
    see Optical spherometer
  front surface, hard, 95
  front surface, soft, 133
  radii of curvature of toric lenses,
    34

Underwater lenses, 125
  air cell lens, 125
  bifocal underwater lens, 126

Vergence, 1
  reduced vergence, 11

Wet cell checking,
  power, *see* Focimeter
  radius, *see* Keratometer *and*
    Optical spherometer

Z value, *see* Edge lift